His Porn, Her Pain

ALSO BY THE AUTHOR

BOOKS

Your Sexual Secrets:
When to Keep Them, When and How to Tell

Ask Me Anything:
Dr. Klein Answers the Sex Questions You'd Love to Ask

Let Me Count the Ways:
Discovering Great Sex Without Intercourse

Beyond Orgasm:
Dare to be Honest About the Sex You Really Want

America's War on Sex:
The Attack on Law, Lust, and Liberty

Sexual Intelligence:
What We Really Want from Sex—and How to Get It

DVDs

Enhancing Porn Literacy in Young People

Talking With Your Kids About Sex

Secrets of Sexual Intelligence

Sexual Intelligence: A New View of Sexual Function & Satisfaction

When Sex Gets Complicated: Infidelity, Pornography, & Cybersex

HIS PORN, HER PAIN

Confronting America's PornPanic
with Honest Talk About Sex

Marty Klein, PhD

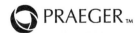

PRAEGER™

An Imprint of ABC-CLIO, LLC

Santa Barbara, California • Denver, Colorado

Copyright © 2016 by Marty Klein, PhD

Library of Congress Cataloging-in-Publication Data

Names: Klein, Marty, author.
Title: His porn, her pain : confronting America's pornpanic with honest talk about sex / Marty Klein, PhD.
Description: Santa Barbara, California : Praeger, 2016. | Includes bibliographical references and index.
Identifiers: LCCN 2016025435 (print) | LCCN 2016035513 (ebook) | ISBN 9781440842863 (hard copy : alk. paper) | ISBN 9781440852213 (pbk.) | ISBN 9781440842870 (ebook)
Subjects: LCSH: Pornography—United States. | Internet pornography—United States. | Sex—United States. | Sexual ethics—United States.
Classification: LCC HQ472.U6 K59 2016 (print) | LCC HQ472.U6 (ebook) | DDC 363.4/70973—dc23
LC record available at https://lccn.loc.gov/2016025435

ISBN: 978-1-4408-4286-3 (hardcover)
ISBN: 978-1-4408-5221-3 (paperback)
EISBN: 978-1-4408-4287-0

20 19 18 17 16   1 2 3 4 5

This book is also available as an eBook.

Praeger
An Imprint of ABC-CLIO, LLC

ABC-CLIO, LLC
130 Cremona Drive, P.O. Box 1911
Santa Barbara, California 93116-1911
www.abc-clio.com

This book is printed on acid-free paper ∞

Manufactured in the United States of America

To John Gagnon, PhD (1931–2016),
Who inspired me to become a sociologist
and
To James Petersen, Playboy *Advisor Emeritus,*
Who taught me how to write about sexuality

CONTENTS

Acknowledgments   ix

FAQs   1

Introduction. "What would happen if America were flooded with free, high-quality pornography?"   5

PART I.   **Context**

Chapter 1. Porn Explodes into America's Homes— Where People Are Very, Very Unprepared   11

Chapter 2. Moral Panics, Sex Panics, and PornPanic   17

Chapter 3. Updating the Panic—The Public Health/ Danger Model   25

PART II.   **Brief Interludes**

Interlude A. The Nature of Sexual Fantasy   37

Interlude B. Deep in the Valley: Going to a Porn Shoot   43

Interlude C. The Myth of Porn's Perfect Bodies   47

Interlude D. Rule 34: What It Says About Your Sexuality   51

Interlude E. No, Mabel, You Don't Have to Compete with Porn Actresses   53

Interlude F.	Guys: More Curiosity and More Empathy Needed	57
Interlude G.	Is There Such a Thing as Gay (or Straight) Porn?	61
Interlude H.	How to Watch a Lot of Porn and Have Good Partner Sex, Too	63
Interlude I.	Does Porn Demean Women?	65
Interlude J.	45 Helpful Things You Can Learn from Porn	69
PART III.	**About You and Yours**	
Chapter 4.	Your Kids and Porn	75
Chapter 5.	Sexting: Who Does It? How Does It Affect Kids?	87
Chapter 6.	Couples' Conflicts About Porn—Innovative Approaches	99
Case A.	Rachel & Jackson: Porn as Infidelity (or, You Thought It = You Did It)	115
Case B.	John & Bora: The Man Who Tried to Communicate Through Porn	123
Case C.	Jevon: The Man Who Tried to Organize the Internet	127
Chapter 7.	How Does Porn Affect Consumers?	133
Chapter 8.	If You're Concerned About Your Involvement with Porn	147
Chapter 9.	Why There's No Such Thing as Porn Addiction— and Why It Matters	159
Chapter 10.	Increasing Porn Literacy and Sexual Intelligence for Therapists, Doctors, and Clergy	175
Epilogue.	A Complicated Consumer Product	185
	Notes	189
	Index	201

ACKNOWLEDGMENTS

"How long did it take you to write the book?" Dozens of people ask this about every book I write, and I never know quite how to answer. I can tell you the day I sat down and started to type. I can tell you the day, months before that, when I sat down, looked out the window, and started thinking about where and how I would start. I can even tell you the day two years before that when I asked my agent about this next book I wanted to write.

What I can't really tell you is how many months and years I've been thinking about this topic: reading about it, corresponding about it, lecturing about it, giving interviews about it, inviting questions about it. And above all, writing about it: four dozen blogposts, two encyclopedia entries, and so on. How long did it take me to write this book? More or less a lifetime. As my reader, would you have it any other way?

I tell you this to underline how important it is for me to be in dialogue with the world about my work. And while a writer necessarily works alone, I am fortunate to have the world's smartest, kindest, and most sex-positive people as friends and colleagues. During lunch after lunch for two years, author Michael Castleman never stopped asking, "Are you going to write the damn book or not?" And when I finally did start writing, he kept being helpful.

Thank you Doug Braun-Harvey, Melissa Fritchle, Paul Joannides, and Kate Sutton, who never tired of talking about this book.

Thank you to the modest and much-loved Mark Kernes for research, legal reporting and illumination, networking, and friendship.

For periodic conversations that challenge me or inspire me—and frequently make us both laugh—thank you Robert Badame, Ellyn Bader, Larry Hedges, Dagmar Herzog, Meg Kaplan, Ian Kerner, Dick Krueger, David Ley, Charles Moser, Margie Nichols, Pete Pearson, Clarissa Smith, and Carol Tavris. Thank you Jim Herriot for endless bike rides with endless, valuable conversations about sexuality.

Thanks to the wonderful men and women of the First Amendment Lawyers Association, including Andy Contiguglia, Bob Corn-Revere, Clyde DeWitt, Jeffrey Douglas, Jennifer Kinsley, Mark Randazza, Lou Sirkin, and Larry Walters. What a privilege it is to have you walk me through the living, breathing labyrinth of American jurisprudence year after year. Your clarity of thought and commitment to principles are both breathtaking.

Thanks to the participants of the Sexnet listserve, moderated by the fearless Michael Bailey. You people are brilliant, generous, intimidating, witty, and aggravating. What a pleasure to wince at your impatient, acid tongues and learn from your passionate, well-disciplined minds.

Thanks to world-class researchers David Finkelhor, Bill Fisher, Mickey Diamond, Neil Malamuth, and Martin Weinberg. Generous colleagues all, talking to you is terrifying, embarrassing, and infinitely enriching.

Thank you to my editor, Debbie Carvalko, who changed my life by buying *America's War on Sex* for Praeger in 2004, and who thus knew exactly how complicated her life would become when she asked me to do another book. Thank you to my agent, Will Lippincott, a gentleman and ferocious advocate: in an industry that seems designed to frustrate writers, you are profoundly supportive.

This is my seventh book with the same wonderful wife. Randi is more than smart and insightful; she's my most important teacher, my co-author in every way imaginable. How else do you suppose I can do what I do?

FAQs

- **Why a book about "His Porn, Her Pain?" What about women's use of porn, or non-heterosexual couples?**

As a therapist, I work with men and women in every conceivable kind of relationship (and non-relationship) arrangement. I rarely hear complaints about porn use in same-gender couples, in polyamorous arrangements, or in open relationships. What every therapist hears about every week is heterosexual women complaining about their male partner's use of pornography. So that's what I decided to write about.

There is, of course, more to say about pornography than just this configuration. Having written seven books, however, I've learned that trying to cover too much in a single book is unwise. I've also learned that no matter how broadly I write, someone will complain that I didn't cover the specific issue that interests them. So I've learned not to try to discuss everything in any single book.

- **Why is there nothing in this book about child pornography?**

Because that is exactly what this book is NOT about. Child pornography is illegal, difficult to find, almost impossible to discover accidentally, and not made by *any* general-use commercial producer. It is made surreptitiously by people who know they are creating illegal images, to be consumed in secret by people who know they are consuming illegal images.

By contrast, almost all of the pornography viewed by consumers in America features adults doing perfectly legal things. It is important that this common, legal activity be discussed without the distraction of the rare, illegal activity to which it bears very little resemblance.

I am *not* saying that there is no child pornography. The production and consumption of these images poses significant legal and social issues. Those issues deserve a book of their own.

• Is this book pro-porn?

No. It's neither pro-porn nor anti-porn. Virtually everyone's life is now touched by pornography, and so the book examines ways we can better understand it, talk about, enjoy it if we wish, and tolerate others enjoying it if we don't.

• Why is there no definition of pornography here? What's yours? What about erotica? How do you define "hard-core"?

In general, "pornography" is sexually explicit materials intended to arouse. Because this is not a legal or medical textbook, I don't think a more precise definition is necessary. "Erotica" is sexy stuff that people don't want to condemn. "Hard-core" used to indicate a clear portrayal of genitalia during sex (intercourse, oral sex, or anal sex); now it mostly is a pejorative, meaning "porn that shows stuff I don't want to see."

• Supporting the availability of porn, how can you call yourself a feminist?

My feminism is the belief that people should have equal civil rights and civic responsibilities regardless of their gender. I also believe that sexuality is an essential, vibrant part of being both a woman and a man. Therefore portraying female and male sexuality—and supporting the enjoyment of each of those by others—is in keeping with feminism.

Feminism does not require that we privilege the pain of some women about porn over the rights of porn consumers, male or female. Feminism does require that we honor the employment choices of adult actresses (and actors) and not patronize them by saying they don't understand what they're doing. Feminism also acknowledges that when women or men face limited economic opportunities—just like when they face a wide range of economic opportunities—different adults value different things in potential jobs.

• Don't you realize that many rapists look at porn?

Yes, rapists look at porn. Tens of millions of non-rapists look at porn as well. In fact, the proportion of rapists and non-rapists who look at porn appears to be about the same.

- **Sure, pornography. But isn't there a limit?**

Pornography doesn't need "limits" any more than any other form of expression. The primary limit needs to be the consent of the participants, which of course would exclude all porn made with minors. The only possible exception to that would be sexy selfies that minors take of themselves and share with peers they trust for private use—a subject that needs far more sober discussion than it is currently getting.

- **Don't you understand the emotional pain people are in about porn?**

Yes I do—in fact, because I'm known as a sex therapist with particular expertise in this area, I work with the issue of pornography and its attendant pain far more than most professionals. I take that pain—whether of consumers or their partners—seriously, and I have devoted a lot of time to thinking of innovative approaches to these difficulties.

Everyone should be troubled by the contemporary idea that only people who are obsessively distraught about others' pain or some social injustice actually notice, care, and understand. I care deeply about the pain some people feel about their own or their partner's porn use—I'm just not willing to say that they're ruined for life, or that they need special arrangements to keep from being triggered, or to exaggerate the mischief that porn causes.

- **Would you want your son or daughter to be a porn actor or actress?**

I would want my child to have lots and lots of occupational choices, from secretary of agriculture to junior high school teacher to struggling novelist to porn performer. I'm dismayed when people have only one very limited way to earn a living, whether it's as a porn performer or working the graveyard shift at 7-Eleven.

- **Why are there 80 kajillion books about how porn ruined the author's life, and only a handful of books like this—doesn't that tell you something?**

It mostly tells me that I'm once again flouting the wisdom of the marketplace in favor of doing work that's meaningful to me.

I'm actually rather disturbed that so many people find their partner's porn use upsetting. In general, I don't think it's porn that ruins people's lives any more than golf or *Downton Abbey*. I do think there are people who either can't or don't want to moderate their own behavior. It's easy to blame the external things to which people migrate, but isn't it more honest to ask a person withdrawing from a relationship to get curious about their passion and their behavior, and ultimately to make different choices?

• At what age do you think kids should watch porn?

Pornography is a product specifically made for adults. It should be watched only by adults, particularly because most young people get virtually no help decoding porn from either parents or sex education. As with many other products designed for adults, however, many people under the age of 18 view porn once, sporadically, or regularly. They deserve adults in their lives to acknowledge this and talk about it in helpful ways.

• What kind of porn do you watch?

As a therapist and social scientist, I never discuss my personal sex life. It would be unprofessional and distracting for readers.

• Why doesn't the book have any illustrations?

To maximize the number of places the book can be displayed, sold and read.

INTRODUCTION: "WHAT WOULD HAPPEN IF AMERICA WERE FLOODED WITH FREE, HIGH-QUALITY PORNOGRAPHY?"

Imagine that you and I were sitting in my backyard during the warm Labor Day weekend in 1999, sharing a nice bottle of Cabernet. "What do you suppose would happen," you might have wondered playfully, "if America were flooded with free, high-quality pornography?"

Now *that* would be an interesting question, and we would have enjoyed speculating about it together for 15 or 20 minutes. Would everyone go on a diet, wanting to look like a porn star? Would everyone get divorced? Would people stop using contraception, or stop having sex with their mate altogether? Would people quit their jobs so they could stay home and watch porn all the time? Would *Playboy* go out of business? Would sexual violence skyrocket? Plummet?

We actually don't need to guess about this, because only 12 months later, that's exactly what happened: broadband Internet brought high-quality pornography into tens of millions of American homes—for free. Within just a few years, the entire country was wired. And watching. Do you know anyone who doesn't use the Internet?

In retrospect, some people call this paradise; others say that all hell broke loose. Either way, Americans are still watching, more than ever. Most of them are loving it. But for millions of men and women, the pain—and the anxiety—are piling up. They're afraid for their marriages, their families, and their country. Some are even afraid for themselves.

The introduction of broadband Internet porn into American homes created what scientists call a "natural experiment." This is the rare chance to empirically observe and study the effects of a specific intervention on a group of people selected by circumstances—the equivalent of being selected at random, making the results very, very informative.

To make it even more interesting, this natural experiment has been replicated in many other countries—with virtually identical results to America's.

So what would happen if America were flooded with free, high-quality pornography?

Now we know. So rather than speculate, we can examine the actual results. By doing so, we could learn quite a bit about human beings, sexuality, and other things. This book is about America's *refusal* to do so—and precisely how this refusal to look at the facts about pornography is hurting marriages, families, kids, and individuals.

We'll also look at the social and political forces at play here. Exactly who has driven this rejection of the facts? As it turns out, there's a lot of money and power to be gained from scaring the hell out of Americans about sexuality in general, and pornography in particular.

* * *

For thousands of years—from pottery to Gutenberg, from rubber to nylon[1]—every new technology has been adapted to sexual purposes. This provokes even more anxiety about the strange new technology, and so these cycles of technological innovation and sexual adaptation are almost always followed by public outrage and fear.

In 1844, for example, Charles Goodyear patented a process for vulcanizing rubber. A few years later the first rubber condoms were produced, and a few years after that, Congress criminalized the mailing of condoms and of condom advertising. They were even condemned by Elizabeth Blackwell, America's first female physician, who predicted they would increase prostitution.

A few years after that, new printing technologies led to a dramatic drop in the price (and therefore to a dramatic increase in availability) of low-brow novels; with the slogan "Would you want your servant or wife reading this?" proper urbanites tried to get the books banned or limited.[2] In the 1920s, the mass spread of cinema soon led to heretofore hidden stories with sexual themes (like prostitution, infidelity, and rape), followed by predictions of moral and sexual disaster that led to the repressive Production Code, under which American movies (and movie-goers) were censored until 1968.

Each time, the outcry generally subsides, and in retrospect usually seems quaint and overblown. If the fear is later vindicated (the birth control pill *did* lead to an increase in non-marital sex), change is ultimately called "inevitable," and eventually dismissed as "progress."

In our own lifetimes we've seen the demonization of then-new erotic commodities and services such as adult bookstores, hotel room porn rentals, thong swimsuits, swingers' clubs, mass-marketed sex toys, and sexting. You might be surprised at how many of these are still criminalized in some states—despite the fact that millions of ordinary people use them regularly. I've testified in several court cases related to these, including the case that attempted to decriminalize the sale of sex toys in Alabama (which failed—it's still illegal).

The pornography industry's early adoption and promotion of the Internet is just the latest example of this 2,000-year-long historical trend. In fact, most people don't realize that it was the pornography industry that built the Internet. The high download speeds, clear resolution, shopping capacity, and synchronized audio-and-video that we take for granted were all pioneered by the pornography industry. Think of that the next time you shop on Amazon for Grandma's birthday gift.

Like all previous technology/sex developments, the public has responded to pornography's development and use of the Internet with massive anxiety and resentment.[3] I now see that concern every week in my therapy office, as spouses, parents, and porn consumers struggle with a dreadful sense that technology has unleashed yet more opportunities for unpredictable, uncontrollable sexual behavior.

The Internet has had a transformative effect on the viewing of pornography. Instead of sullenly trudging to a dingy downtown theater, or being embarrassed at a neighborhood video rental store, people can now consume porn in complete privacy—not only from strangers and neighbors, but even within their own home. And they can do so whenever they like, without having to purchase or rent something in advance.

However the lack of privacy (and availability) limited porn-watching in the past, the Internet has blown those limits away. Now people can watch as much as they like, whenever they like, choosing whatever niche genres they want. This radically enhanced availability is a much bigger change than the fact that porn depictions are now more varied and intense than they were before the Internet.

The result of super-availability? Huge numbers of men watch. More women watch than ever before. Teens and pre-teens watch—on their smartphones. People watch at work, even (or especially) when their workplace is the military.[4] A few people now watch in public—on airplanes, in libraries, and in moving cars. Scientists in Montreal recently tried to do a study of porn consumption using a control group—but they couldn't find enough college-age men who had never looked at porn.[5]

Some might surmise that all this porn was welcomed as a great addition to Americans' sexual expression. But all this broadband porn was not dropped into a society eagerly waiting for it. Or ready for it. In fact, it was dropped into a society that had significant difficulties regarding sexuality. One could have easily predicted that it would have an explosive, and not entirely welcome, impact.

PART I

Context

Chapter One

PORN EXPLODES INTO AMERICA'S HOMES—WHERE PEOPLE ARE VERY, VERY UNPREPARED

In and before the 1950s, pornography had historically been attacked as "immoral." During the Cold War years, some members of Congress even declared it was part of a Communist plot to weaken the character of America's youth and husbands.[1]

Religious figures like Billy Graham and Fulton Sheen had enormous national followings, enjoying regular audiences with sitting presidents. Their portfolio was protecting America's morals, and pornography was a key battleground.

This immorality crusade defined pornography as broadly as possible; in 1956, for example, the influential Legion of Decency condemned the film *Baby Doll* ("a steamy tale of two Southern rivals and a sensuous virgin") for its "carnal suggestiveness." Francis Cardinal Spellman denounced the film from the pulpit of St. Patrick's Cathedral before it opened, saying it had been "responsibly judged to be evil in concept" and would "exert an immoral and corrupting influence on those who see it"; he called for all Catholics to refrain from seeing the film "under pain of sin." And this was a high-concept film, written by Tennessee Williams, directed by Elia Kazan, and starring Karl Malden.

But morals change; even more important, the *role* of morals changes as well. In the 1960s, recreational drugs, rock music, and films imported from Europe, along with the Vietnam War and the Watergate scandal, challenged the landscape of American morality. The birth control pill changed the definition of what "good" girls do. A president was eventually impeached as madly lustful—although not convicted.

Political battles about abortion raged, with anti-choice activists justifying the eventual murder of 11 physicians and other clinic personnel (and the attempted murder of 26 others[2]) as moral. A battle also raged about an alleged "homosexual agenda,"[3] and whether "morality" precluded or required withholding a variety of common rights (family hospital visits, tax breaks, adoption, etc.) from gay people.

Planes were hijacked and flown into American buildings, and a new kind of "them" enacted *their* morality by targeting American lives in Boston, Chattanooga, and elsewhere. Catholic priests—seen by millions as the last bastion of rock-solid, old-fashioned morality—were exposed as having coerced thousands of children into sexual activity.[4]

Finally, in 2003, the Supreme Court decided *Lawrence v. Texas.*[5] In addition to decriminalizing same-gender sexual behavior, the majority wrote that an alleged majoritarian morality was not a sufficient basis for a law regulating private behavior.[6] The Court had turned 180 degrees in only 17 years, when it had ruled that morality *was* a legitimate basis for depriving citizens of their rights to privacy and sexual choices in their own homes.[7] Clearly, the *place* of "morality" in American public life—however "morality" was defined—had changed forever.

People and organizations attempting to control American sexual expression, used to doing it through the time-honored vehicle of promoting "morality" and preventing "immorality," were stuck. To maintain their political power, social prestige, and financial standing, what were they to do?

* * *

Recall that before broadband Internet became freely available in 2000, pornography was only semi-legal. *Playboy* and *Penthouse* could not be openly displayed in many outlets, such as 7-Elevens; adult bookstores operated in a twilight zone, just one zealous prosecutor away from financially ruinous arrests and years of imprisonment.[8] Sending "obscene" videos through the mail was illegal, and if a prosecutor could simply find 12 jurors willing to say a video was worthless trash, its makers and marketers lost all protection of the First Amendment. I have testified in such cases as an expert witness, looking on helplessly when defendants were jailed.

Although millions of people were using adult porn on the eve of broadband's introduction, the federal government had spent decades pursuing, prosecuting, and jailing Americans for creating adult porn or for selling it to other adults.

The high point of this campaign was when born-again Christian President George W. Bush directed the Department of Justice to create a new task force to go after those in the adult pornography industry. For such victimless crimes, hundreds of people languished in jail for many years.

If we understand what happened when broadband Internet brought porn into everyone's home less than 20 years ago, it's easier to understand why we're at such a complete standstill in our ability to deal with it now—and why there's so much anxiety, resentment, secrecy, and confusion about porn today.

DISRUPTIVE TECHNOLOGIES

By definition, no society is ever ready for disruptive technologies, and the environment into which an innovation arrives shapes the way it will be received. (Of course, history doesn't say much about innovations that don't get accepted, and simply die quietly—you know, like cashmere dental floss.)

For example, when photography was invented around the time of the Civil War, most soldiers were away from home for the very first time. Similarly, most wives were without their husbands for the first time. Women used the new technology to create and send erotic postcards to encourage their sweethearts to be careful (so they would return), which men treasured while trying to survive an overwhelming new kind of industrialized slaughter.[9]

A century later, the birth control pill arrived at a time of great social ferment, when sexual mores were changing and college dorm rules were being liberalized. In 1968, I myself lived in one of America's first co-ed dorms, at one of the first universities whose health service dispensed these magic pills that suddenly made sex a lot safer.

The social context into which broadband pornography entered tens of millions of American homes in the first years of the 21st century? The United States was an enormous tangle of sex problems. If it had been a person, it would have needed medication; if it had been a couple, it would have required marriage counseling; if it had been a teenager, it would have been grounded, sent to its room without dessert.

But it was a country. And this country had an array of sex problems bigger than *Seinfeld*'s George at his most neurotic:

- School sex education was driven by the abstinence model—its federally mandated goal was preventing kids from having sex, not educating them about it, or teaching them how to make good decisions about it. Congress specifically refused to require that sex education be medically accurate. The policy, not surprisingly, was a dismal failure.[10]
- The country was reeling from a frightening HIV/AIDS epidemic. Often treated as a disease caused by promiscuity or perversion rather than by a virus, many religious and political leaders said HIV proved that sex is dangerous. Many communities such as the Catholic Church simply refused to discuss it, or to discuss prevention strategies involving condoms.[11]

- Congress and Presidents Bush I and Clinton had been trying to censor the Internet since its commercialization in the 1990s; states including New York, Michigan, and Arizona tried, but were defeated in federal court. The reaction to the scary new Internet included calls for mandatory filters on computers in libraries, schools, airports, universities, state offices, and elsewhere.

  For example, students and staff using University of Arkansas computers cannot access my website because of automatic filtering software. The reason is presumably because the content is about sexuality. I say "presumably" because filtering software is proprietary; even when the public pays for it, companies are under no obligation to reveal what's in it, or how it works, or how users are protected from arbitrary or political decisions made by the filtering companies.[12]

- America had the highest rate of unintended pregnancy in the industrialized world. This was especially true of teenagers.

- By many accounts, America was the land of sexual dissatisfaction. Books, TV shows, and magazines continually documented Americans' low rates of marital sex and sexual satisfaction. At the same time, half of marriages experienced infidelity.

- As the most religious country in the industrialized world, there were many taboos against talking about sex honestly, or even acknowledging one's true sexuality to oneself. Most organized religion was actively encouraging people to feel guilty about their sexuality—their desires, arousal patterns, preferences, fantasies. The Catholic Church had reaffirmed its opposition to all effective methods of contraception. Mainstream Christianity led the opposition to effective sex education. It still presented premarital virginity as an ideal for all women—demanding that millions of women second-guess their own sexual decision-making.

- The disease of "sex addiction" had been invented 15 years prior. Despite its lack of recognition by professional organizations like the American Psychiatric Association, it was accepted as a legitimate disease by much of the lay public, religious leaders, and moral entrepreneurs. Well-known celebrity sex addicts like Michael Douglas were popular in the news, and media "therapists" like TV's Dr. Phil and radio's Dr. Laura shamed them—and their audiences.

- Fear of homosexuality had reached a boiling point. President Bill Clinton had recently signed the Defense of Marriage Act, putting the federal government's full weight into the battle to prevent gays from supposedly destroying heterosexual marriage. At the very same time, gay people were being dishonorably discharged from the military every month, for fear that they would use shower time to seduce straight soldiers (recorded instances of this: 0).

- President Bill Clinton was impeached—impeached!—for perjury and obstruction of justice related to his sexual indiscretions (a trial that was arguably America's first reality show). The impeachment failed, despite Independent Prosecutor Kenneth Starr's 1998 investigation. The Starr Report mentioned oral sex exactly 92 times, a phrase that everyone in America soon had on their lips—usually with a perfectly American blend of disdain and titillation.[13]

In short, when broadband brought unlimited free, high-quality pornography to America, the country was obsessed with sex—both with controlling it, and, ironically, with experiencing it in various forms (for example, via voyeurism, sex work, porn, and infidelity). And here was a new technology that facilitated virtual sexual experiences with few limits. Depending on one's perspective, it was either a dream or a nightmare—the classic American agonized struggle over sexuality.

Introducing the option of unlimited, free, high-quality, highly varied pornography into this volatile mix of ignorance, fear, anger, sexual dissatisfaction, curiosity, and sexual cravings led to some absolutely predictable results. These included:

- Tens of millions of people used porn the second it was easy.
- Many people got overinvolved with it—and couldn't speak with anyone about this. Most recovered and stabilized their viewing, the same way that most people eventually recover from HBO bingeing after they get accustomed to having access to so many great shows. A small number of people continue watching in unhealthy amounts or in unhealthy ways.
- Because porn use was pathologized (and porn was demonized), lots of reasonable consumers felt isolated, ashamed, and confused. Whatever the impact of porn-watching on consumers, the impact of this marginalization is larger.
- Few couples had the communication skills they needed to deal with hurt or conflict about porn. To avoid this, many consumers hid or lied about their porn use, which had worse effects on their relationship than the porn use itself.
- Most parents refused to talk with their kids about it. Kids certainly weren't going to bring it up, so kids were left to deal with this on their own.
- Lacking both sex education and adult discussions of sex, young people turned hungrily to porn to learn about sex. Consuming an adult product without adult guidance, many young people became confused about their experience. Much of what they thought they learned was inaccurate.
- Almost overnight, couples and families found themselves dealing with anxiety or conflict about pornography. As both people and their devices became

more creative, usage increased; within months of broadband's introducing porn into every home, new patients came to my office focused on problems with porn. Similarly, the therapists I trained were suddenly clamoring for advice on how to deal with the porn-related problems they were seeing.

- Psychologists, physicians, and pastoral counselors were unprepared to deal with the enormous volume of porn use.
- Within this chaotic, anxious environment, no politician or civic leader was willing to suggest a rational, fact-based public policy discussion. The result was a set of laws and policies that still damage Americans—for example, by criminalizing teen sexting.

Yes, introducing an enormous new range of sexual options into an environment of fear, anxiety, shame, and ignorance led to a huge psychological, cultural, and political mess. And while consumers and non-consumers dealt with it in their own personal ways, moral entrepreneurs promoted a damaging moral panic—a PornPanic—that was absolutely predictable.

That mess—that PornPanic—is still with us, stronger than ever. It drives public policy, influences parenting, supplies the media's narratives, and encourages millions of marital quarrels every year. That's why understanding it matters.

Chapter Two

MORAL PANICS, SEX PANICS, AND PORNPANIC

Today's PornPanic is part of a long, troubling American tradition of moral panics about sexuality. Like clockwork, every few years we can see the public's ongoing sexual obsession with degeneracy, pollution, profligacy, debauchery, and inversions of social order.[1]

For starters, what are moral panics?

Moral panics are symbolic crusades against artificial threats inflated by the media and other public figures. They are a response to perceived threats to social order and to future generations (like the panic over the "homosexual agenda"). Moral entrepreneurs whip up fear and outrage disproportionate to any actual danger, with lurid stories of depravity and innocent victimhood (like the 2015 panic over the videos allegedly showing Planned Parenthood "harvesting" fetus parts). The result is a volatile emotional climate in which people energize into constituencies united to defeat a common social threat (the way anti-porn feminists are now working with the anti-women's-rights religious right). Facts and logic become incidental to the "real" story of deviance, conspiracy, or betrayal (as with today's anti-vaccination conspiracy theorists), and anyone challenging the crowd's panic response is punished publicly (as with scathing attacks on lifelong gender rights activists Dan Savage and Germaine Greer, for not being sufficiently "transgender-friendly").

"Moral panics," says social psychologist Gil Herdt, "are the natural disasters of human society, like tsunamis and hurricanes. They present a crisis . . . that threatens the well-being of individuals and communities."[2]

An example of a moral panic is the 1950s hysteria about the damaging effects of comic books on children. In Fredric Wertham's 1954 book *Seduction of the Innocent*, his amateurish "research" concluded that comic books led to antisocial behavior among young readers.[3] His solution? Make them illegal for kids under 15. In response, parents dragged their children to public burnings of comic books; censorship and other restrictions gutted the comics industry, while the Senate convened hearings about juvenile delinquency and comic books.[4] Fearing government suppression, the industry created the Comics Code Authority (CCA), which enforced "modest" dress codes on characters; enforced bans on words like *zombie* and on characters like vampires; and insisted that police had to be portrayed positively, and divorce negatively.

Other contemporary moral panics include the marijuana scare of the 1960s ("reefer madness"); the persistent rumors of snuff films in the 1970s following the gruesome Charles Manson murders; the backward masking scare (that playing rock albums backwards would yield messages encouraging devil worship) in the early 1980s; the Dungeons & Dragons scare soon after, as evangelical Christians claimed role-playing games led to suicide or mental illness; and today's anti-vaccination movement, which claims childhood vaccinations cause autism, regardless of nearly unanimous scientific opinion to the contrary.

Let's look back over the last one-and-a-half centuries of sexually-oriented moral panics.

Only a few years ago, gay people were ostracized as mentally ill, predatory, and profoundly Other. They were blamed for AIDS (for example, by the Westboro Baptist Church) and for undermining heterosexual marriage (remember state after state passing Defense of Marriage legislation?). As would-be presidential candidate Michele Bachmann put it in 2014 and again in 2015, gays "want to abolish age of consent laws, so adults could freely prey on little children."[5,6]

A decade before that, America went through convulsions about children at risk of being kidnapped, raped, and killed (exceedingly rare, according to the FBI)[7]; in response, Congress passed Megan's Law in 1996, which created the world's largest database of registered sex offenders, whose definition expands every year.[8]

Before that, Surgeon General Joycelyn Elders had commented that teaching students about masturbation was acceptable in school sex education; by the time her opponents finished indoctrinating the media, her comments were reported as "young children should be taught how to masturbate," for which she quickly lost her job.

Before that, it was a panic about satanic ritual abuse, a supposed conspiracy that kidnapped children for black magic ceremonies, prostitution, pornography, forced incest, and rape.

Before that, it was the new rock 'n' roll music; frightened communities lit bonfires of records, "suggestive" songs were banned from radio, and Ed Sullivan censored Elvis Presley's historic live television appearance from the waist down.[9] Before that, it was the first publication of Kinsey's data on human sexual behavior,[10] which was accused of promoting moral depravity.

Before that, Congress held hearings about the sexual dangers posed by comic books, and before that, people feared the sexual seditiousness of the new medium of radio. Before that, people feared Irish, Italian, and other (mostly Catholic and Jewish) immigrant groups' irrational, barely-controlled lust.

Before that, it was the masturbation panic during the turn of the 20th century, when loving, terrified, middle-class parents actually chained their children's hands at bedtime to prevent "self-abuse." Before that, those same middle-class people were solemnly instructed that the new (and criminalized) contraceptive devices would hurt their bodies, marriages, and souls.

Before that, it was supposedly oversexed black men who had to be lynched before they preyed on white Southern women (who, it was feared, secretly desired these oversexed and overendowed men).

Today's panic about broadband porn (what I call PornPanic)—complete with "modern" ideas about brain imaging, the biology of addiction, lab studies of rape ideology, and rumors of the overwhelmingly violent, homogenous content of Internet porn—is just the latest turn of the moral panic wheel. In the foreseeable future, we will see these ideas judged silly and old fashioned, much as we think of leeches, blood-letting, exorcisms, insulin shock therapy, and gay conversion therapy today.

When it comes to sexuality, America seems to always be sliding into, recovering from, or gripped by one moral panic or another. Going back to the Salem Witch Trials, our centuries-long tradition of conceptualizing sexuality as a profound danger requiring vigilance and regulation[11] was the fertile consciousness on which the seeds of broadband Internet pornography began to fall in 2000. It launched the current moral panic that demonizes porn, marginalizes its consumers, lies about its content, speculates wildly about its effects, invents new diseases it causes, willfully misinterprets its spirit and artistic conventions, and uses it as the stand-in for everything scary and confusing about the digital age.

This tradition made the new pornography a sitting duck for those who patrol our social order. It has remained so to this day—**even as the country has shifted from an immorality critique of pornography to a public health critique of pornography.**

Today, the Internet is used by at least 87 percent of the entire American population, including children.[12] It's hard to recall that in 1999 only a third of U.S. adults were Internet users—typically spending very little time on it, using slow dial-up modems to connect.

That is, in the year 2000, most of America knew nothing about the Internet of the 1990s, when people started wrestling with the astounding new Internet of the future—and broadband porn flooded the country at the very same time. It was as if a small number of people were learning how to swim, and then every home was given a speedboat.

In fact, here's a similar story of intertwined technological and social change. On my first trip to China in 2011, I noticed that many Chinese drivers were extremely nervous, and they didn't know how to use all the knobs and features on their car's dashboard. I was puzzled until I realized that a majority of China's drivers had grown up in a home where no one owned or even drove a car. Rather abruptly, life had been completely reorganized in a way that no one could predict or control.

Because the new Chinese middle class had bought luxuries like cars only recently, there were of course plenty of accidents. More important, however, was the amount of anxiety and confusion that developed from the sudden introduction of private cars and private driving: Is it safe to drive in the rain or at night? Are other drivers looking at me while I drive? Does driving cause cancer? Is it high status or low status if my wife drives? Should I wash my car every time I drive it? Is it better to live near a highway, or away from it? Is it OK to litter while I drive? If I can take the bus somewhere, how do I decide whether to drive instead? If I drive, should I pick up strangers at bus stops along the way?

Unlike Americans, most Chinese adults have no childhood memories of riding in their parents' car, talking with their parents about driving, or talking with their friends about riding in their parents' cars. In 2011 (and still true in much of the country), people in China were simultaneously learning how to drive *and* how to integrate cars and highways into their lives.

Today, we cannot minimize the fact that **in 2000 the American public was confronted with round-the-clock free porn at the same time they were learning about the most profound technological innovation of the last 5,000 years.** Clearly, dealing with anything new while learning how to integrate the new high-speed Internet into our lives would be complicated—all the more so with something taboo like porn.[13]

So while the country didn't exactly come to a standstill in 2000, it did rather quickly plunge into a PornPanic. The people and organizations who led the way did so because of money, power, personal agonies, or because they were true believers. Or some of each.

* * *

As America awoke to the 21st century and broadband Internet, it had all the ingredients needed for a moral panic about pornography. It still does, involving many of the same people and organizations riding the PornPanic gravy train. Most important was the confusion, anxiety, and sense of overwhelm that high-speed Internet brought. Pornography was only a part of that—a significant one, but part of a larger sense of cultural overwhelm that still affects us as we continue wrestling with this increasingly powerful new Internet.

This sudden PornPain was (and continues to be) masterfully exploited. It continues to be nourished by existing morality groups that leaped at the chance to renew their relevance. Groups like Morality in Media (rebranded with a new title focusing on danger, not morality) and Citizens for Community Values gave themselves new missions, such as eliminating pay-per-view pornography in hotel rooms (they succeeded dramatically in Ohio, and helped change the corporate policies of Omni and Marriott). Without any data whatsoever, radically anti-sex, self-proclaimed "feminists" like Andrea Dworkin and Patrick Trueman linked adult pornography to sexual violence and sex trafficking. Those myths are stronger today than ever.

President George W. Bush himself added to the panic, unleashing the Department of Justice to go after "hard-core pornographers" to—of course— "protect our children." He urged the DOJ to go after pornography because it was allegedly dangerous, not merely distasteful or immoral. The Attorney General encouraged people to believe that Internet porn was somehow related to Internet predators, thus directly endangering kids; he made few distinctions between adult porn and child porn, which frightened parents and communities even more.

Several idiosyncratic features of American society help(ed) fan the flames of PornPanic.

1. An aggressive Internet filtering software industry

In a perfect example of capitalism at work (every entrepreneur's mission: create or exaggerate a need, then sell a product to address it), an industry quickly arose in the late 1990s to address parents' confusion about their kids using the Internet. It fanned their anxiety to a fever pitch, describing the Internet as a jungle of deviant pornography and a haven for predators— essentially an open sewer of toxic material. At the same time, the industry described their products as perfect solutions that would create that blessed, oft-pursued and rarely-achieved state—safety. Here's a typical marketing line for one company: *"An open Internet is unsafe for children, and parenting in this digital age is difficult. We provide tools for parents to control unwanted content and [to] provide a safe Internet for your family."*[14]

Whether they bought these products or not, parents, legislators, educators, and workplace decision-makers got the message: The Internet is a dangerous source of sexual material and lust.

Not at all paradoxically, in keeping with basic capitalist strategies, these companies selling safety and security fanned the public's fear and anxiety— the PornPanic.[15]

2. Lack of training of therapists, social workers, clergy, or physicians, who were suddenly asked to deal with this new issue.

Historically, clinicians dealing with concerns like mental health, relationships, and parenting get almost no training in human sexuality. You can be trained as a marriage counselor without ever hearing the words vibrator or kissing. You can do pastoral counseling for 20 years without uttering the words clitoris or fantasy. And almost no doctor hears the word masturbation during their training or subsequent continuing education. While there are of course exceptions, this group of professionals has historically been poorly informed and rather conservative about sexuality.

So when laypeople had questions about the new pornography and the challenges it presented to them as consumers, couples, and parents, their traditional sources of professional advice and comfort were mostly clueless. They fell back on their old paradigms regarding gender, intimacy, and sexuality, which weren't necessarily helpful. To make things worse, the clinical professions are historically slow to adopt new non-clinical technologies (such as fax machines and mobile phones), and they were slow to become familiar with the digital world and the Internet.

To this day, clinicians know very little about the actual ecology of people's porn use (indeed, about people's sex lives), and they don't usually feel comfortable discussing it. They rely on the same PornPanic tropes as the general public: porn addiction, porn as violent and demeaning to women, porn as harmful to kids, porn as undermining otherwise good marriages, and selfish husbands with victimized wives.

When the mass media want expert voices in their articles, interviews, or panels, these are the professionals to whom they turn. They reinforce, rather than allay, the PornPanic.

3. Misuses of porn

There are always people who misuse every technology, old or new. Cars have been with us way over a century, and people still drive drunk. We've had a dozen kinds of contraception available for years, and people still get pregnant unintentionally. We've had radio for generations, and people still listen to Rush Limbaugh. Commercial flight eventually led to 9/11, as well as to hellholes like Newark and Heathrow airports.

And so of course many people misused the new Internet, surfing endlessly, buying pointless stuff on eBay, communicating compulsively with everyone they'd ever met, playing round after round of *Tetris, World of Warcraft*, and games on Xbox (apparently not infrequently at work).

Predictably, some people misused the new porn. Teens with smartphones emulated it by creating porn of themselves, sharing it with boyfriends, girlfriends, or others they wanted to impress. Some people distributed photos they'd received in private, as a form of revenge when relationships went bad. Others even posted them on websites and demanded payment for taking them down.[16] Most disturbingly, some people used the Internet to circulate pictures of adult-child sex. One hears of the Deep Web, filled with illegal sites involving child pornography and sex trafficking.

With the new Internet and the new porn paired with such activities— impulsive teens flaunting their sexuality, psychopaths getting revenge on former lovers, child porn producers peddling their forbidden wares—of course people were judgmental and scared. It served to validate the warnings of the moral entrepreneurs. And of course the media played up these stories to make them seem far more common than they actually were.

So that's how America got here, and that's what keeps us here: gripped by a PornPanic, complete with exaggerated dangers, new diseases and social pollutants, willful denial of fact, identified scapegoat, multiple cheerleaders with media access feeding the fear and anger, guilt by invented association ("porn creates demand for trafficking" is the latest), and moral entrepreneurs demanding political, legal, fiscal, and cultural action (everything except research) on the alleged threat.

Chapter Three

UPDATING THE PANIC—THE PUBLIC HEALTH/DANGER MODEL

How, then, could moral entrepreneurs like Morality in Media, Concerned Women for America, Parents Television Council, and Family Research Council continue to oppose pornography in a world in which the public consensus on "morality" and "immorality" was unraveling, and the concepts themselves had become less relevant, less motivational, and less discussed by the public?

How could such groups express moral disapproval, and demand social policy based on morality without basing this on opposition to immorality? And how could they energize and expand the base of the anti-porn movement just as pornography (carried by broadband Internet) was arriving in everyone's home, looking as if it might become as American as apple pie?

Such a crisis was also a tremendous marketing opportunity. The response was reinventing pornography as a Public Health Menace. Only the most extreme people talk about the immorality of watching porn anymore; instead, almost everyone who opposes porn now talks about how dangerous its use and existence are to consumers and to society.

As social scientist Alan McKee notes, when religious shaming goes out of vogue, "sin" is simply replaced with "unhealthy."

And so government, activists, decency groups (both old and new) and most churches[1] switched the anti-porn narrative from "porn is immoral" (vaguely bad for *users*) to "porn is dangerous" (concretely bad for *everyone*). Americans started hearing that viewing pornography caused consumers to rape and molest. And that it ruined marriages, damaged brains, stole erections, harmed teens, supported crime, scarred children, perverted adult desires, distorted men's ideas about "normal" sex, damaged the actors and actresses who made it, led men to dehumanize women, and created addiction. This justified the demands, continuing to this day, that porn be restricted or even criminalized.

On the eve of his execution in 1989, convicted mass murderer Ted Bundy said that violent porn made him kill his many victims. James Dobson, executive director of Focus on the Family, proceeded to popularize this interview as "proof" of porn's pernicious effects, and demanded government action.[2] Ridiculously, the views of a deranged psychopath are *still* being quoted as insight about public policy.[3]

Porn thus became a legitimate civic concern for whole new constituencies that weren't being moved (or were even turned off) by the "immorality" argument, such as feminists, psychologists, addictionologists, criminal justice professionals, domestic violence activists, and anti-trafficking advocates.

* * *

As the increasingly sophisticated and increasingly ubiquitous Internet brought free, high-quality pornography to an increasing percentage of the American public, a number of groups and individuals became increasingly distressed. Although some of them—traditional allies, such as the Catholic Church and right-wing morality groups—did coordinate their response, many others acted on their own, for their own separate reasons. Nevertheless, the net effect was a broad attack on pornography by a variety of civic players—including some traditional opponents, such as feminists and the Catholic Church, brought together in a de facto alliance against a shared enemy.

Essentially, an ad hoc array of civic propaganda militias launched a full-scale war on the use of a legal product by 50 million people. That war continues today.

The key weapon in that war was the successful transformation of the primary cultural narrative about pornography. Porn use has been changed from a behavior that is immoral (for oneself) to a behavior that is dangerous (to everyone). Porn consumers are no longer seen as compromising primarily themselves, but rather as endangering everyone around them, from loved ones to neighbors to complete strangers.

Behavior (porn use) heretofore considered *private* has been reconceptualized as *public* (despite the fact that it is still done in private). Like other private sexual behaviors such as sodomy, marital swinging, sadomasochism, reading "obscene" books, and going to strip clubs, porn use has been "public-ized" by social fiat.[4]

Everyone who follows current affairs has seen the importance of controlling the social narrative of contentious events or political struggles. Look at the power of these contrasting labels in a wide range of issues:

- global warming vs. climate change
- gay marriage vs. marriage equality
- pro-life vs. anti-choice (and pro-abortion vs. pro-choice)
- lack of will power vs. alcoholism
- mini-van vs. light truck
- child abuse vs. no-nonsense discipline
- illegal aliens vs. undocumented workers
- homosexual agenda vs. civil rights for all
- redevelopment vs. eminent domain property seizure
- self-abuse vs. masturbation vs. self-pleasuring

In our instantaneously interconnected world, controlling the narrative of what's going on is fully as important as controlling what's going on.

As America continues to grapple with the chaotic, exponentially growing world of the Internet, anyone can identify themselves as a stakeholder regarding its supposed effects. Concerned about pornography, a wide range of groups has done so: addictionologists, feminists, psychologists, religious leaders, child advocates, government, sexual violence activists, media scholars, morality groups, and law enforcement, to name a few.[5] This has led to odd political alliances; for example, conservative feminists working with anti-choice activists, Internet safety activists working with anti-technology home school advocates, or addiction therapists working with child safety advocates.

Acting mostly independently, each group uses its own tactics. In no particular order, these include:

- Inventing the disease of "porn addiction," blatantly redefining the word "addiction" without any clinical rigor
- Declaring porn use a threat to marriage without any studies comparing marriages in which porn is and isn't used
- Resurrecting 30-year-old laboratory studies of porn's effects on college student attitudes without acknowledging what, exactly, they measured and found
- Citing tiny, exploratory neuroscience studies and implying they indicate that porn use affects long-term brain function
- Inventing the disease "pornography-induced erectile dysfunction" (PIED), despite the lack of data showing an increase in erection problems in users
- Defining porn use as "infidelity" despite most couples having no prior agreement about whether either will use porn during the marriage
- Defining porn as "demeaning to women" despite most porn showing women in states of desire and pleasure, being fulfilled by a willing partner; various activists actually object to the use of vibrators, the focus on female "pleasure," and depictions of female "enthusiasm"[6]

- Portraying porn actresses as emotionally damaged people (without any evidence) further exploited by an uncaring industry
- Saying the production and consumption of porn encourages sex trafficking, despite a lack of data indicating this
- Saying that porn use is bad for teens' brain development, using extremely hypothetical models
- Conflating the effects of watching a lot of porn with the effects of high Internet and smartphone use
- Ignoring the historic data on the incidence of sexual dissatisfaction in marriage
- Ignoring government data on the decrease in rates of sexual violence, teen pregnancy, divorce, and other social pathologies since broadband made porn accessible to everyone, all the time
- Distorting the typical content of porn, claiming it's all dramatically violent

Note that virtually none of these arguments or strategies was used to oppose the creation or use of pornography as recently as 40 years ago.

The cumulative effect of these independent actions has been to create a coherent narrative of porn as a consumer product dangerous to both its users and to everyone else. The combined effect of these multiple, synergistic narratives is to create the impression that only people who are selfish, sick, desperate, lost, obsessed, oblivious, or criminal use the product.

And so 50 million people—three times the number of people who watched the World Series last year, more than the entire African-American population of the United States—has had their private recreation pathologized, demonized, and marginalized. Their private recreation is now a Public Health Danger.

Like all moral panics, today's PornPanic is accompanied by massive amounts of misinformation repeated endlessly. If you live in America, you have heard the following myths not once or twice, but over and over. And from multiple sources: a religious figure here, a conservative feminist there, a media psychologist agreeing with a "victim" of porn, a child welfare or anti-trafficking advocate solemnly interviewed without challenge. When the public hears the same message from such a diversity of sources, echoing each other's false estimates, it becomes hard to imagine that they're all wrong. But the following common myths are *factually incorrect.*[7]

Myths About Porn:
The Nuts and Bolts of the Public Danger Model of Pornography

- Myth: Porn is mostly violent and "misogynist."
- Fact: It's mostly non-violent. It shows female sexual passion (e.g., women loving cunnilingus or fellatio), which some people define as misogynist.

In any other context, problematizing female passion is considered unacceptable. The anti-porn assumption that depicting women as enjoying sex is misogynist should be seen as misogynist, too.

- Myth: Watching porn causes erection problems, especially in young men.
- Fact: There's no data showing there are more erection problems now than before 2000, and no data that if there are more erection problems, they're caused by watching pornography.

- Myth: Porn destroys enjoyable, intimate relationships.
- Fact: There's no data that this occurs. There are people in relationships whose stability depends on ignoring or hiding sexual dissatisfaction; when porn viewing becomes an issue in a couple, it may appear as if porn viewing is responsible for the sexual dissatisfaction or relationship problems. No one, however, leaves a good intimate relationship for pictures of pretty young women (or men).

- Myth: Most men hide their porn-watching from their partner because they know they're doing something wrong.
- Fact: Most men who watch porn don't think they're doing something wrong. When they hide their porn-watching it's because they believe they have to protect their wives' feelings, or because their wives have forbidden them from watching, so they must resort to secrecy—instead of challenging the unilateral prohibition, which could lead to conversations extremely uncomfortable for both parties.

- Myth: Only a man would enjoy porn; women simply don't like it.
- Fact: Millions of women watch porn alone; as many as 10 million watch with their partner. Over 100 million copies of the *Fifty Shades of Grey* trilogy have been purchased—virtually all by women.[8] It may lack photos, but yes, with explicit descriptions of sex, sexual feelings, and sexual bodies, this book is porn, porn, porn.

- Myth: Watching adult porn leads to watching kiddie porn.
- Fact: There is no evidence for this. In fact, the audiences for the two products have almost no overlap. Most adults find the idea of watching kiddie porn so repulsive that nothing could get them near it, certainly neither enjoyment of nor boredom with their current adult porn. The adult (legal) porn industry does not create kiddie (illegal) porn, and therefore doesn't market it to consumers.

- Myth: Porn is all about men's sexuality and men's pleasure.
- Fact: This is contradicted by watching any random three minutes of almost all pornography featuring women. Women are generally portrayed as enjoying whatever activities in which they're involved. Their characters almost always desire the sex they have, and almost always orgasm. If they

provide their partner(s) with pleasure, they are usually shown enjoying it. Male viewers enjoy consuming depictions of women's sexuality, ranging across women's desire, arousal, pleasure, satisfaction, curiosity, communication, seduction, fantasy, preferences, domination, submission, and anatomy.

- Myth: Watching porn encourages violence against women.
- Fact: The rate of sexual violence toward women in America has *declined* since the rate of porn consumption dramatically *increased*.

The early studies on whether porn use encourages sexual violence was collected primarily from college students in a laboratory and focused primarily on self-reported attitudes toward women, rather than actual behavior (without ever studying any actual links between the two). Later studies used open-ended questions about actual porn use and actual male-female behavior; this research found little effect of porn use on sexual violence.

- Myth: Neuroscience proves that watching porn can damage the brain (especially in the young) and even cause porn addiction.
- Fact: The burgeoning field of psych-neuroscience reports similar changes in the brains of people cuddling puppies, enjoying sunsets, and watching porn. Neuroscientists do *not* claim that watching porn does *anything*— rather, this is the work of activists citing ambiguous reports of neuroscientists, which laypeople aren't trained to evaluate.

The new disease of porn addiction is simply an updated version of the disease of sex addiction, created in the 1980s by prison addictionologist Patrick Carnes. Without the hallmarks of true addiction—changes in physical functioning, need for increased dosing, withdrawal symptoms, and continuing the activity when it isn't enjoyable—it's hard to take this claim seriously.

* * *

Misinformation like this creates a sense of distance and of porn's Otherness, despite porn's ubiquity. And the more people continue to feel porn is Other, the more that distance continues, which is critical for maintaining the Public Danger narrative of the PornPanic.

Through it all, the voice of porn consumers is conspicuously absent.

So how do we account for the persistent myths about pornography and the demonization of this product, a product used by more people than the number of adult Americans who drink soda every day?[9] How do we account for the fear, the rage, the insistence that this product is pernicious when people are confronted with contrary evidence all the time—i.e., their own porn-watching mate doesn't murder anyone, demean women, molest children, or look at child porn?

The anti-porn industry is strong and still growing. A quick review of Amazon.com, for example, reveals dozens of books written about the cultural and personal disasters caused by porn in just the last few years. And a wide range of websites attacks porn's alleged harms, ranging from xxxchurch.com to nofap.com to pornharms.com—none involving a credentialed professional. This outpouring is both the result of and continuing contribution to a moral panic, similar to the ones we've seen in America periodically since before the founding of the Republic.

The transformation of opposition to porn from the immorality model to the Public Danger model matters for several reasons. It gives concerned sweethearts a new, worrisome explanation for their mate's behavior, while it gives angry wives and girlfriends justification for saying their partners are doing something wrong (as opposed to "I don't like it"). It encourages parents to worry rather than talk to their kids.

We'll see how this looks in real people's lives in Part III. It really does matter what narratives we're marinating in.

* * *

Here's an unusually clear picture of the Public Danger model of pornography, a model that invites *everyone* to mobilize against porn. In January 2016, the state legislature of Utah passed a resolution declaring pornography a Public Health Crisis (see next page). It's an amazing document, asserting over a dozen false "facts"; attributing causation to pornography that isn't documented; describing supposed social problems in ideological terms; and calling for young people to not abandon marriage.

The resolution ends with the faux compassionate, ". . . overcoming pornography's harms is beyond the capability of the afflicted individual to address alone."

To the extent that the Utah resolution names serious problems in society (such as misinformation about sexuality and violence toward women), those should be addressed via sex education, family conversations, porn literacy, well-informed therapists and school clinics, and parenting classes. Alas, the resolution suggests none of these. In fact, within weeks of passing this resolution, the very same legislature voted down a bill that would allow comprehensive sex education in Utah schools—a low-cost intervention scientifically proven to reduce many of the problems the resolution claims need addressing.

* * *

What is the only reasonable response to this fact-free declaration, this self-righteous pile of hellfire judgments ("deviant sexual arousal"?), this deliberate mischaracterization of private recreation from the state with the highest per capita use of porn in the United States?

Figure 3.1 shows what has happened since the introduction of free, high-quality pornography into virtually every home in America.

CONCURRENT RESOLUTION ON THE PUBLIC HEALTH CRISIS
STATE OF UTAH 2016 GENERAL SESSION

Be it resolved by the Legislature of the state of Utah, the Governor concurring therein:

WHEREAS, pornography is creating a public health crisis;

WHEREAS, pornography perpetuates a sexually toxic environment;

WHEREAS, efforts to prevent pornography exposure and addiction, to educate individuals and families concerning its harms, and to develop recovery programs must be addressed systemically in ways that hold broader influences accountable;

WHEREAS, pornography is contributing to the hypersexualization of teens, and even prepubescent children, in our society;

WHEREAS, due to advances in technology and the universal availability of the Internet, young children are exposed to what used to be referred to as hard core, but is now considered mainstream, pornography at an alarming rate;

WHEREAS, the average age of exposure to pornography is now 11 to 12 years of age;

WHEREAS, this early exposure is leading to low self-esteem and body image disorders, an increase in problematic sexual activity at younger ages, and an increased desire among adolescents to engage in risky sexual behavior;

WHEREAS, exposure to pornography often serves as children's and youths' sex education and shapes their sexual templates;

WHEREAS, because pornography treats women as objects and commodities for the viewer's use, it teaches girls they are to be used and teaches boys to be users;

WHEREAS, pornography normalizes violence and abuse of women and children;

WHEREAS, pornography treats women and children as objects and often depicts rape and abuse as if they are harmless;

WHEREAS, pornography equates violence towards women and children with sex and pain with pleasure, which increases the demand for sex trafficking, prostitution, child sexual abuse images, and child pornography;

WHEREAS, potential detrimental effects on pornography's users can impact brain development and functioning, contribute to emotional and medical illnesses, shape deviant sexual arousal, and lead to difficulty in forming or maintaining intimate relationships, as well as problematic or harmful sexual behaviors and addiction;

WHEREAS, recent research indicates that pornography is potentially biologically addictive, which means the user requires more novelty, often in the form of more shocking material, in order to be satisfied;

WHEREAS, this biological addiction leads to increasing themes of risky sexual behaviors, extreme degradation, violence, and child sexual abuse images and child pornography;

WHEREAS, pornography use is linked to lessening desire in young men to marry, dissatisfaction in marriage, and infidelity;

WHEREAS, this link demonstrates that pornography has a detrimental effect on the family unit; and

WHEREAS, overcoming pornography's harms is beyond the capability of the afflicted individual to address alone:

NOW, THEREFORE, BE IT RESOLVED that the Legislature of the state of Utah, the Governor concurring therein, recognizes that pornography is a public health hazard leading to a broad spectrum of individual and public health impacts and societal harms.

BE IT FURTHER RESOLVED that the Legislature and the Governor recognize the need for education, prevention, research, and policy change at the community and societal level in order to address the pornography epidemic that is harming the people of our state and nation.

Figure 3.1
Pornography Availability and Decrease of Social Problems

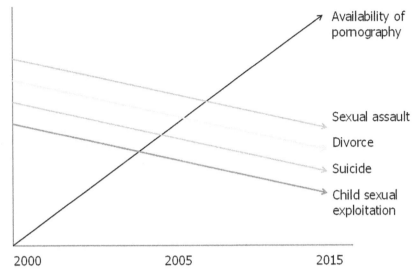

Pornography → Social Problems?
(schematic)

Availability of pornography

Sexual assault

Divorce

Suicide

Child sexual exploitation

2000   2005   2015

Source: Author

Yes, the rates of rape, divorce, suicide, and child sexual exploitation have all *decreased* since porn flooded America.

So why is Utah (*and* Concerned Women for America, *and* the National Center for Sexual Exploitation, *and* Focus on the Family, *and* the Family Research Council, *and* Covenant Eyes, *and* so many others) so committed to fighting the wrong thing?

PART II

Brief Interludes

Interlude A

THE NATURE OF SEXUAL FANTASY

Although virtually everyone has a voyeuristic streak (hello, *People Magazine? Entertainment Tonight?*), at the very same time there are things most of us don't want to know: the handsome guy who picks his nose. The perfect woman with rotten produce in her fridge. The wise therapist who loves guns, bullfighting, and Fritos. We don't really want to know.

The same is true about others' sexual fantasies. On the one hand, we're eager to see behind the erotic curtain—what kind of underwear, what kind of positions, what kind of orgasmic sounds? On the other, the potential for ick is everywhere: you get off imagining *what*? I'll defend your right to imagine it (or watch it) until I die, but really, dude—you get erect thinking about that? Disgusting!

And that's part of the issue about ubiquitous, 24/7 Internet porn: it documents what everyone's fantasies are, and invites us to confront what used to be people's private sexual imagination. Some of us are pretty dismayed by others' fantasies.

Because the totality of porn, like the totality of, say, shoes or beer, is a statement of what others find interesting. They wouldn't make your favorite shoe if you were the only one who bought it. They wouldn't make your favorite beer if you were the only one who ordered it. And they wouldn't make your favorite porn—that is, cater to your particular fantasy—if you were the only one who found it hot. So just like the shoe department at Nordstrom or Target is a living inventory of the kinds of shoes people like, porn is a similar living document, a compendium of human sexual fantasies—from the popular to the esoteric.

The difference is that, unlike Nordstrom or Target, pornography is a compendium of fantasy—not *desire*, but *fantasy*.

We have a love–hate relationship with others' fantasies: we want to know—until we don't want to know. And then it's too late. How am I ever going to forget I've seen *that* porn? Or forget that some of my fellow humans think that's hot? We shouldn't blame porn when our voyeurism leads us to places we wish we hadn't gone. Rather, we should smile at the naiveté we didn't realize we had about the enormous range of human sexual fantasies. It's a reminder to love our fellow creatures, whose bizarre fantasies are just like ours, except different.

Another issue regarding porn is the common misunderstanding that our fantasies have meaning—specifically, that that's who we really are and what we really desire in life. And so with a feminist who gets hot imagining being spanked or the gentle guy who gets hot imagining spanking, both feel guilty and ashamed.

But fantasy does *not* equal desire.

Many anti-porn crusaders (and even smart people like the authors of *A Billion Wicked Thoughts*[1]) make the mistake of assuming that what arouses people on video or on a page indicates what they want to do in real life. But that's wrong: people watch *Matrix* or *The Terminator* and don't go crashing their cars; people watch *RoboCop* or *Natural Born Killers* and don't go out and kill; people read *Fifty Shades* and don't go looking for someone to tie them up; heck, people watch Olympic curling and they don't go out and curl.

We know that in general, fantasy has limited predictive value. Why imagine that's different when the fantasy's subject is sexuality?

The panic about the truth of others' sexual fantasies depends on the persistent myth that enjoying a fantasy is the same thing as desiring it in real life. If that were true, millions of our neighbors would be punching their bosses, sleeping with their brothers-in-law, selling their homes to start over in Boise, or urinating on the very next TSA guard that hassles them.

One of the ways healthy people cope with the pressures and complicated decision-making of adulthood is fantasy. We watch *Star Wars* and *Star Trek*, *CSI* and *Grey's Anatomy*, *Batman* and *Wonder Woman*. We watch NASCAR and Wimbledon. And we daydream, "If only that were me . . . if only I had the chance. . . ." But we don't expect to actually find ourselves on Daytona or Center Court, and generally wouldn't accept the invitation if it were offered.

Some people say sexual fantasies have meaning—that, like dreams, they're a psychologically safe place where we're working out our issues.[2] While that might be true for some people some of the time, I don't think that dynamic is at all universal. People find things hot for infinitely varied and impenetrable reasons.

But even if you want to say that fantasies have meaning, decoding that meaning for any given person is impossible. Male college student–female college professor? It could be acceptance by Mom, a desire to surrender, nostalgia for feelings from 2nd grade, yearning for a skillful partner, rejection of younger women who have been rejecting you, desire for older sister, imagining increased prestige from peers.

Two men kissing? It could be acceptance by Dad, same-gender curiosity, discomfort with women, feeling masculine, or imagining two big penises in those two male mouths.

Watching a man being cuckolded by his wife? It could be guilt about being sexual, an impulse of generosity, imagining being more sexually adequate, surrendering to an adult container, or giving away something that you don't really value.

So you never know. I think we're better off assuming that any given sexual fantasy is an opaque combination of cultural memes, biographical vagaries, visual punch, serendipity, and the phase of the moon divided by what you had for dinner. What percentage of each? We have no idea. Ultimately, it's more important to accept and enjoy our fantasies than to understand or decode them.

The answer to the question of "why that porn rather than this" for most people most of the time is "um, I don't know—I just do." It's similar to explaining why you prefer the ice cream flavor you do—which most people can't do, either. If you give me 10 flavors and ask me to rank-order them, I can—but don't ask me how I do it, other than "I just like this more than that." Ditto porn—most people can rank-order a dozen videos, but can't tell you why, other than to describe them. ("This one has big boobs, that one doesn't." "Why do I like big boobs better? I don't know.")

Regardless of why you like the specific things you do, why do you look at/fantasize/read (i.e., consume) what turns you on? Why do people in general like to watch sexy images, read sexy words, look at sexy people?

- It's fun to look at naked women and/or men who look like you'd like them to (regardless of what that is—and it is *not* always the social definition of perfect).
- It's fun to watch people having sex, which one almost never gets to see in real life.
- It's fun to imagine doing what those people do, feeling, seeing, hearing, tasting, and smelling what they do.
- It's fun to imagine having things you don't have, or will never have.
- It's fun to imagine having things you've lost.
- It's fun to imagine knowing what to do (and how to do it) if you only had the chance.

- It's fun to imagine being accepted, desired, dominated, or dominating.
- It's fun to imagine being seen the way you see yourself—or the way you'd like to see yourself.
- It's fun to imagine enjoying things that definitely won't, absolutely can't, certainly couldn't, and better not happen.
- It's fun to imagine doing things that you wouldn't do in a million years. That's exactly what fantasy is for—to "have" experiences without any consequences whatsoever.

Each year, Pornhub, one of the world's largest porn sites, reports statistics on popular search terms and viewed video categories.[3] Last year it reported on over 32 billion video views in the United States alone. The most popular search terms include lesbian, stepmom, stepsister, and ebony/black. The most viewed categories are teen, lesbian, and throughout the South, ebony.

Some women are shocked, *shocked*, that their partners fantasize, and what they fantasize about—young, beautiful, enthusiastic partners. Or taboo power dynamics, whether with the young, the old, or in-between. The data on the nation's sexual fantasies was also accompanied by a lot of hand-wringing and predictions of evil. OMG—fantasies about teens!

The concern about porn and teens is amusing, and as completely ignorant of history as only Americans can be. Teens have been the center of human erotic attraction since the beginning of time. Evolutionarily, they're perfect for mating. And their bodies are as close to perfect as human bodies get. *Of course* they're attractive to us today—they were attractive in Shakespeare's time, in the Middle Ages, in Jesus's time, and in Roman, Greek, Persian, and Hittite civilization before that. Nothing novel about it.

You do know that until only about 100 years ago there was a special word for teen girls, right? "Wives." Abigail Adams was a teen when she married John, as was Marie Antoinette when she married Louis XVI. Shakespeare's Juliet is described as 13, normal for Renaissance women who married as soon as they reached puberty to overcome the era's high infant mortality rate. Cleopatra ascended the Egyptian throne as a teen, the most desired *woman* on two continents. No man would have been admonished for fantasizing about her—as we read the words Shakespeare puts in Anthony's mouth, it appears he did, too.

But let's be consistent. Because Pornhub's top search terms also include lesbian, MILF, and stepmom, where is the outcry about porn consumers at risk for turning into, or desiring, lesbians? Or all the porn watchers suddenly turning toward older women, thereby depriving younger women of the relationships they deserve? Don't forget granny porn—does its popularity predict an abandonment of all women under 50?

Many women are even more baffled by the non-teen fantasies men apparently have (according to the data on porn site visits): older or old women; lactating or menstruating women; men; ordinary-looking people; groups; domination, submission, deception, even violence; and, of course, every fetish the human mind can conceive or struggle with (shoes, cigarettes, gloves, urine, crushing bugs, even—*gasp*—white cotton panties).

The thing about *these* fantasies is that it's harder for a woman to imagine her guy truly wanting these experiences (which of course he generally doesn't). And so the question of "why do you deliberately watch that when you want to get aroused" becomes more urgent. To an anxious, misinformed woman, it starts to seem that her partner is less known, more complex, possibly "kinkier" (meaning less known and more complex). What *else* does he imagine that she doesn't know about or understand? Being confronted by a loved one's actual sexual fantasies is to lose your innocence—regardless of how sophisticated your own sexuality is.

Interlude B

DEEP IN THE VALLEY:
GOING TO A PORN SHOOT

I've been on movie sets and I've been on network TV, and I've spoken with people working at almost every job in the porn industry. But in all these years I'd never watched a porn film being made.

A few years ago while in Los Angeles, I finally accepted an invitation. After lunch, I drove out to the San Fernando Valley, parked in a neighborhood of modest homes and small warehouses, and walked into the studio of Brash Films. I spent about two hours there, watching and occasionally chatting. Everyone involved made me feel welcome.

The most interesting thing I have to say about it all is—nothing.

But maybe not for the reasons you think.

Sooner or later, watching the same people having sex is repetitive and boring—unless, of course, you're adding to it via fantasy, imagination, arousal, and voyeurism. I didn't do much of that, because I was there working (yeah, I know—tough gig). So yes, watching the shoot did reduce the sex (along with the filming itself) to a technical craft. She used her left hand when the camera needed it, even though she's right-handed. He stopped right in the middle of licking her when a bit of his sweat dripped into a bowl of fruit.

Some people condemn how watching porn at home supposedly does the same thing—it reduces sex to "mechanics." But the critical difference between watching a film being made and watching it at home is what the consumer brings to the experience. And that transforms the "mechanics" into something stimulating.

Those who say that watching porn reduces sex to mechanics aren't adding anything to the film. Nothing positive, that's for sure.

This is the same dynamic when consuming any media—whether it's *Seinfeld*, or *The Mona Lisa*, or *Star Wars*. In fact, both Bach and the Beatles are just noise unless the listener adds something to them. Ever listen to Chinese classical music and think, "This isn't music"? I went to China last spring, and sure enough, most of their tunes sounded like noise to me—because I didn't know what to add to the sound to turn it into what I recognize as "music." On the other hand, the Chinese architecture, although certainly not Western, looked like art to me, because I was able to add something to it. But I couldn't make the Chinese music sound like "music," so it sounded like noise. The same is true with Coltrane or Miles Davis, if you're not conversant with their hum. To be truthful, I'm not wild about their stuff, either.

But back in L.A., what I brought to the porn shoot was nothing. And because of the situation, I was perfectly willing to have a bland, non-erotic experience.

What a consumer brings to a porn film is imagination, privacy, a little time, maybe lube or a toy. And that gives the images meaning—erotic meaning. When anti-porn crusaders take the same film and add fear, anger, and a sense of helplessness, they also give the images meaning—but distinctly un-sexy ones (such as "exploitation" and "immorality"). So:

Porn + nothing = neutral meaning
Porn + fear + loneliness + anger = negative meaning
Porn + privacy + time + imagination = positive meaning

* * *

In all, it was just like being on any other movie set: a bunch of working people wearing t-shirts and shorts (except for Her, Him, and Him), intensely concentrating and cooperating for short bursts of time—and then stopping to adjust a light, mop a brow, snip a loose thread, or find some damn beeping that only the sound guy can hear. Then another short burst of activity, stopping when a scene is completed. Or when an actor really needs to pee.

Of course, the focus was on the people having sex. Her underwear was gorgeous, and she had exactly the body it was designed for. The guys had abs and muscles on top of their abs and muscles, and pretty fair penises, too. But what I admired most about all the bodies was their backs. You gotta have a strong back to thrust and thrust and keep thrusting. You gotta have a strong back to twist around and service a guy at each end, changing positions without missing a beat.

I imagined what these people do in their spare time—a little bit of sex, and a lot of time at the gym. And some Pilates, definitely.

* * *

I wasn't on the porn set on a political mission—in fact, I had no agenda at all except to just be open to whatever happened. But I finally couldn't help asking myself—what is there to complain about here? Crew, actors, actresses: they're all adults, they're all getting paid, they all know exactly what they're doing. No one's exploited, no one's been tricked into thinking they're making Art. They know they're not working with Pixar or Spielberg, Natalie Portman or the Coen Brothers. And they're also not working the breakfast shift at Starbuck's.

They're making a living. Like most working stiffs, they're not brilliant, they're good enough.

I saw a few orgasms (perhaps), spoke with a couple of tech people, and thanked the director. Several people on break thanked me for coming. I gave them a copy of my book *America's War on Sex*, which they admired.

They have their craft, I have mine. Different in some ways, not so different in others.

* * *

Reminiscing about my trip to a porn shoot reminded me of the wonderful coffee-table book *American Ecstasy*.[1] It's sexy, funny, artistic, thought-provoking. What else could you ask for?

OK, here's something else: its photographer/author Barbara Nitke raised hell when she (and others) sued the federal government a decade ago, challenging the constitutionality of the Communications Decency Act, which criminalized the posting of "obscene" content on the Internet.

But let's get back to her marvelous new book.

In 1973, Nitke's husband Herb produced the historic film *The Devil in Miss Jones*, launching the Golden Age of Porn. Nine years later, as the era was coming to a close, Nitke was hired to shoot publicity stills as porn films were being shot. The industry was filled with energetic young people straight out of film school, all creating a new genre of movie. Many of the performers were creative and self-aware as well.

As Nitke recalls, "Every time [I started a new shoot], I had a fresh feeling of running away to join the circus. I had a ringside seat at the greatest show on earth."

With this book *American Ecstasy*, we do, too.

The photos feature garter belts and boom mikes; naked men and women patiently awaiting the perfect placement of a spotlight; exhausted, gorgeous women catching a nap between takes, hair mussed. There's an astonishing photo of a nude 27-year-old Nina Hartley straddling Damian Cashmere's face—and talking to director Henri Pachard.

All the while, Nitke is telling us what is was like for her—and this woman can write. She's funny, she's insightful, she's compassionate, she's melancholy. A gifted storyteller, she recalls the hard work, the frustration, the triumphs—and the humanity of everyone concerned. She generously adds commentary by the giants of the era. Nina Hartley says some pretty smart things about being in the business. So does Candida Royalle. So do a lot of the men and women involved in creating the images we've been living with for decades. They're the subterranean explorers for a society that has a never-ending thirst for what they do—while marginalizing and damning them for doing it.

American Ecstasy is simultaneously three books. There are the sexy, compelling, sometimes surprising photographs. There's the writing by both Nitke and the various participants. And there's the juxtaposition of the photos and words, which gives heightened resonance to each other. We can read Ron Jeremy's thoughts ("It's a wonderful life . . . but once in a while, I hate to think that this is all I've done . . . it all ended in my being a porn actor, and that's as far as I got.") while looking at a photo of him enraptured with the girl of our dreams. Candida Royalle talks about her years of needing rape fantasies in order to get real satisfaction.

Whether through picture or story, the book features dozens of fascinating people: Sharon Mitchell, Joey Silvera, Nina Hartley, Ron Jeremy, and others. Together they've been involved in hundreds of millions of American orgasms. Millions of hours of American ecstasy.

The production of this book is simply fantastic. The binding, the heavy paper, the voluptuous color all combine to bring these images and this era to life. With all due to respect to Kindles and iPads, if you like actual *books*, you will love this *book*.

Some people say a picture is worth a thousand words. As an author, I've always said that a word is worth a thousand pictures. With Nitke's work, we don't have to choose. Combining words and pictures, she documents an era brimming with outlaw eroticism, fearless experimentation, and youthful innocence. In this unique way she enriches our perspective on something that has become, for many of us, quite mundane. And she entertains us at the same time.

It's a great accomplishment, definitely worth the price, and a highly recommended treat for yourself, or for someone you love.

Interlude C

THE MYTH OF PORN'S PERFECT BODIES

Among the complaints I repeatedly hear about porn is that it features perfect female bodies, which supposedly makes male consumers lose interest in normal, imperfect bodies. Normal imperfect bodies, of course, are what most men are limited to in real life.

People who allege that porn features only perfect bodies (including uniform, perfect labia) are almost always unfamiliar with actual porn. Porn consumers don't describe porn that way, because it simply isn't true.

Sure, many porn consumers seek out and enjoy conventionally perfect bodies—young, unblemished, wrinkle-free, incredibly round where they're round, as smooth and firm as polished teak where they're smooth and firm.

But an enormous percentage of Internet porn features adult bodies very different from that. If you don't watch porn you wouldn't know this. But if you watch adult porn, you know what's out there, including:

- Amateur porn: Porn posted by non-professionals, usually made in their homes or hotel rooms. These men and women look like you and me—unless, of course, you look like Brad Pitt or Scarlett Johansson.

Amateur porn not only features the non-gorgeous, it sometimes features the downright average-looking. And that's what consumers of amateur porn apparently often want—regular people looking regular, doing sexual things. It's the genuine enthusiasm that these consumers love, combined with the idea that the film could have been made by neighbors just down the street.

Now if only we could get those neighbors to vacuum the living room before making their next video.

- Non-silicone, often non-perky: Critics who claim that every porn actress is puffed up with silicone are full of, um, hot air. While the eerily perfect silicone look has lots of fans, so does the natural look.

Many top porn actresses feature exactly what they grew on their own, glorious imperfections and all. And some have less than they used to—whether they're called hangers, droopers, suckers, or saggers, there's an audience for breasts that are definitely not youthfully perky. What a great country—whatever breast type you like (including small and extra-small), there's porn made exactly for you.

- Fetish: While many porn sites feature videos for the mainstream, others cater to niche markets. Fetish sites aren't for everyone, but one by one they feature everything you can imagine, and plenty you don't: women who don't shave their legs, women on their periods, women with giant clitorises, women with bald heads, women amputees, women who are lactating, women wearing diapers, women a little overweight, a lot overweight, and so overweight they have trouble navigating a doorway.

No Plain Janes need apply here.

Why do some consumers like to wank to pictures of pregnant women or women finger-painting with their menstrual blood? People who enjoy it answer exactly the same as everyone else describing their favorite visual arousal: "I dunno, it just works for me." That's the same answer you give when asked why you prefer the flavor of fruit juice that you do, right?

- Old: There's mommy porn, granny porn, grandpa porn, in-law porn, mature porn. That's a lot of gray hair.

Some crusaders say that watching videos of old people being sexual is even more disgusting than watching "normal" (still objectionable) porn. But these days we all believe it's OK for older people to be sexual, right? In fact, every evening TV commercials show older people getting ready for sex—with Viagra, Cialis, and Levitra, not to mention medications for pain and overactive bladder. So how are videos of their sexuality any more perverted than videos of young adults having sex?

The "decency" critics want to have it both ways—they demonize porn for featuring unrealistically beautiful young actresses, and then they cringe when porn features more normal-looking middle-aged or older actors and actresses.

* * *

So what does this all mean?

First, people who don't know porn should stop talking about what porn shows. For critics who say, "But I don't want to watch that crap," fine, don't watch it—but then you don't get to be a critic. If you insist on being an ignorant critic, at least preface every third sentence you say with, "Of course, I don't know what actual porn is like, because I haven't really seen any."

Second, people surprised with the real content of porn should ask themselves—if it isn't just the perfect bodies, what else do people want from porn? Why do they watch stuff that I wouldn't watch in a million years if I wanted to be aroused?

That's where things get interesting, because humans watch and get excited by an incredibly wide range of sexually explicit material.

So why does our human family love consuming images of things they don't necessarily want to do themselves? Consider common video choices: straight men like to watch men fellating men. Inhibited people like to watch orgies. Assertive women like to watch submissive women.

We are a perverse species.

Different people watch porn for different reasons. We shouldn't be surprised that different people like different kinds of porn, including porn that you or I might find boring, disgusting, stupid, or way too much like our first marriage.

If we thought of porn the way we think of everything else—TV, novels, clothes, kitchen appliances—we would have predicted this. In porn, as in most things, American consumers have a wide range of choices, and they vote with their eyeballs. Every eyeball likes perfect images. Intriguingly, every person with eyeballs imagines perfection differently.

If a decency crusader doesn't watch porn, and thinks that people engage with porn differently than they engage with everything else in their lives, he or she wouldn't—couldn't—imagine this.

And if a decency crusader knows nothing about everyday life, he or she could easily overlook the simple fact that all of us are surrounded by gorgeous bodies—at work, at the grocery store, in the airport, at the gym, on the street—and have to figure out how to stay interested in our imperfectly bodied mate at home. Porn is the least of that problem, which has existed in the West since the Greeks and Romans.

Interlude D

RULE 34: WHAT IT SAYS ABOUT YOUR SEXUALITY

Rule 34 is: If it exists, or you can imagine it, there is porn (or sexualized examples) of it. No exceptions. (And Rule 34a: If it doesn't exist, it soon will.)

Why does Rule 34 deserve its own interlude here? Because it summarizes everything about sexuality.

It says that human sexual fantasy is limitless. It says that anything can be eroticized, can be arousing, can be life-affirming. It reminds us that any ideas we have about what constitutes normal sex are about us, not about sex. I'm always telling patients, "Don't blame sex for your ideas about sex."

Rule 34 reminds us exactly what pornography is: a library of human eroticism. Pornography is a celebration of how humans can stretch their erotic imagination—sometimes in ways that disturb you or me. Nevertheless, pornography celebrates the erotic imagination *beyond* specific content. Like the ability to imagine the future, and the knowledge that we're going to die, the enormous range of pornography is uniquely human.

Rule 34 also reminds us that people don't necessarily want to do what they fantasize about. Sex with Kramer, George, and Jerry at the same time? Sex with a dolphin? Sex with someone about to be guillotined for stealing a loaf of bread? Sex with your grandmother at high noon on Times Square? A threesome with Batman and Robin?

Rule 34 also reminds us of the coin's other side—that none of us can imagine the entire range of human eroticism. That should keep us humble. It's somewhat like a gourmet travelling to a far-off, isolated country and discovering the locals eat something he never considered food—say, fried worms.

The issue isn't so much whether or not the gourmet wants to eat fried worms; rather, it's the idea that there's "food" that he never considered to be food. And if that's true about fried worms, about how many other "foods" might that also be true?

Rule 34 shows that we're all knitted together in an erotic brotherhood and sisterhood. If the human project of eroticism is bigger than both you and me, your turn-on and my turn-on that appear so different from each other are really small parts of a much bigger whole. And there are others who are into your turn-on (which I find so exotic), and there are others—perhaps many others—who think my turn-on is so very exotic.

Imagine travelling to another country whose customs may be unfamiliar. We go to Italy and see adults and children topless together on the same beach. We go to India and see cows on the street. We go to Vietnam and see old women doing manual labor on construction sites. We go to Denmark and see men and women nude in a sauna together. We go to Russia and learn we have to bribe taxi drivers with Marlboros if we want them to pick us up.

International travel teaches us about our own customs: when I return from a trip I've always learned something about the way *we* do things, because I've been to a place where they don't do that. I learn that my way isn't the right way, it's just my way. No matter how much I prefer it, no matter how much it's right for me, it's just my way, not the right way.

Rule 34 helps us understand that about sexuality. Your porn isn't right, it's just your porn. That goes for No Porn, and Gentle Porn, too: it isn't right, it's just your way. And that goes for our sexuality in general—our way isn't the right way, it's just our way. A good sexual relationship involves people whose respective ways mesh: one person expands their vocabulary, or both do, or one narrows theirs, or both do. As long as people can fit together with dignity and celebration (um, there's *my* values again), it doesn't matter what they do.

Rule 34: Everyone else is different from you. But governments, religions, and activists try to whitewash almost every kind of sexuality except the version of which they approve. As biologist Mickey Diamond says, nature loves variety; unfortunately, society hates it.

Interlude E

NO, MABEL, YOU DON'T HAVE TO COMPETE WITH PORN ACTRESSES

One of the objections that some women have to their partners watching porn is, "I can't compete with the women in those videos."

The idea that a woman has to compete with the women or activities in porn films is an unfortunate misunderstanding.

Now, some women feel they have to compete with mainstream celebrities like Selena Gomez and Beyoncé (and before that, with Marilyn Monroe and Sharon Stone, and before that, with Helen of Troy). That's a fool's errand that no one should attempt. These are professionals; do not attempt to do their job in your home.

If you're smart enough to realize you can't (and don't need to) compete with JLo or JLaw, why would you feel compelled to compete with Candye Kisses or Rosie Cheex?

While making superficial comparisons in life is inevitable, most men know that porn is a fantasy, not a documentary. No one actually expects his girlfriend to pay the pizza delivery guy with oral sex, and no grownup really expects his partner to look or act like a porn star. Like the NFL and Cirque du Soleil, people in porn are selected for their unusual bodies. *Very* unusual bodies.

Sadly, sometimes it's women, not their men, who are comparing themselves with porn stars. Ladies, you're not competing with a real person, you're attempting to compete with a cinematic character—who has the benefit of lighting, editing, a fictional partner with unlimited energy and desire, and a script instructing her to defy gravity while moaning on cue.

You can't compete with that character any more than your man can compete with the James Bond character, the Captain Kirk character, or the Sherlock Holmes character.

Perhaps a glance at "supermodels without makeup" will help put things into perspective.[1] Ladies, unless you're a porn actress with professionals working on your makeup, hair, and lighting, you won't look like a porn actress when you have sex. And without editing equipment in your bedroom, you won't sound like one, either.

By the way, let's be honest—plenty of women love to consume images of gorgeous females, too. Who else is the audience for *People Magazine*, *E! News*, and those award-show red carpet previews? And please don't say you're interested in "fashion" or "style" (or "news")—the audience's interest is in beautiful women wearing clothes that reveal more than they cover. Admit it—aren't you a little disappointed when some famous babe shows up in a pantsuit or something that hides her cleavage?

(Note: Shouts of "sexism!" do not constitute a thoughtful critique here. No one ogling Leonardo DiCaprio or Matthew McConaughey is thinking "What a fine actor" or "What an expressive artist." No—eyeballing these guys is the same activity as eyeballing Sofia Vergara. Can't we just admit it and get on with our fantasies?)

That said, plenty of porn features women who are not conventionally beautiful. There's amateur porn, granny porn, saggy-boobs porn, and obese porn, to name a few. People who view such things are looking for something other than perfect bodies. They may enjoy watching ordinary-looking people doing ordinary sexual things. They almost certainly enjoy the actresses' erotic enthusiasm, whether it's been scripted for professionals or it's authentic from amateurs.

If there's any way your man compares you to porn, it's most likely about enthusiasm—which for almost all men trumps a perfect body any time. Good news: this means your less-than-perfect body doesn't disqualify you in bed.

When women are convinced that their partners are thinking about porn stars while having sex with them, I ask how they know this. During sex does he call you the wrong name, does he seem a million miles away, does he keep talking dirty even when you've repeatedly asked him not to? Most women answer no. Instead of evidence, they say, "Why would he focus on my lumpy body during sex when he could be thinking about Ophelia Rump, who's perfectly round and firm?"

Why would he? What about feeling desired, touching and being touched, kissing, nibbling, smelling, pleasing someone else, and feeling part of the ongoing human erotic parade? Sex with Mary FiveFingers while watching porn may provide more perfect stimulation and a more reliable orgasm, but when it comes to sex, friction isn't everything.

So if your question is, "Why would he focus on me during sex?," you may need to look at your sexual self-esteem. I'm very sympathetic if you can't imagine why he'd rather focus on the live, imperfect naked woman he has with him rather than a maybe-perfect-looking body in a movie.

You might want to check how much your self-consciousness or despair about your body is undermining your mutual sexual enjoyment. It's not like you're going to wake up next week with the perfect body or boundless energy of a 24-year-old (unless you're 24 right now), so you both need to figure out how to eroticize the conventional body of a person your age, in your condition.

At work, at the supermarket, in the airport, the world is full of beautiful bodies, male and female. Porn or no porn, every man and woman has to figure out how to feel OK with themselves when they aren't as good-looking as others.

And how to feel OK when they don't have as much money as others, don't have jobs as prestigious as others, or don't have kids as smart as others. This is the fundamental existential task of all people who want to enjoy life, and porn didn't invent it.

* * *

Memo to any guy who resentfully tells a woman, "Why can't you look like the women in porn," or, "Why can't you do what the women in porn do?": Dude, the "women in porn" are *acting*. They're following scripts designed to get you hot. Very few people do those things in real life, and very few people look like that in real life. They're like the characters in *Lord of the Rings*.

If you want your partner to be more enthusiastic or adventurous about sex, criticizing her and comparing her to fictional characters—like Wonder Woman or The Girl With The Dragon Tattoo—is guaranteed to fail miserably.

Interlude F

GUYS: MORE CURIOSITY AND MORE EMPATHY NEEDED

I don't hear many gay or lesbian couples quarrel about pornography. But if you're a man in a sexual relationship with a woman, and she complains about your porn-watching, you need to be curious. If she seems unreasonable to you, you need to be even more curious: What could possibly bother her about something that seems so harmless to you? Regardless of what you do about it, you have a responsibility to know the answer to that question really, really well.

As a sex therapist, and when taking questions on the radio and at my lectures, I hear a lot of women concerned about their guy's porn-watching:

"He has a secret life."
"I feel left out."
"It's something I just don't understand."
"I feel inadequate compared to porn."
"I'm afraid he watches really creepy stuff."
"I trust him less."
"I'm afraid he's hooked."
"He's so defensive about it."

While some women do catastrophize over this domestic situation, everyone is entitled to their feelings. And I'm afraid that in many cases I'm not impressed with men's responses to concerns like these.

Gentlemen, you're not going to talk her out of her distress. You're not going to ridicule her out of it, bully her out of it, logic her out of it, or even sweet-talk her out of it. You might get her to talk about it less, but you won't get her to feel less.

So stop trying. You may be frustrated, guy, but stop trying to change how she feels. Instead, do the opposite. Encourage your partner to talk about herself. How does she feel (as opposed to what she thinks) when she reflects on you watching porn? Have her feelings about it changed over time? How does she believe it affects your sexual relationship? How does she feel about your sexual relationship in general? Are her feelings more about you watching porn or about you masturbating?

Further, what does she imagine you watch, what does she imagine you feel while you watch, what does she image you think about your experiences? What's her theory about why you want to continue watching despite her discomfort?

Curiosity can be a beautiful thing.

You don't have to agree with her about any of this, but knowing more about how she feels and what she imagines is crucial to the two of you resolving this chronic ache. The process of feeling more understood can itself be healing for her, just as the process of understanding her better will be valuable for you. The more you see her as a person in pain (rather than as someone hassling you over your unimportant private thing), the closer you'll feel and the more emotionally flexible you'll both be. That's when you're most likely to solve a problem together, rather than each partner suggesting solutions that mostly suit one of you.

When a couple is in conflict, each person's instinct is usually the same: "You need to understand me better. Let me explain things again." If both people are pursuing that path simultaneously, the exchange isn't likely to be productive. If instead one or both people are committed to understanding the other person better, there's a chance they can make progress on resolving the conflict.

So if your partner reveals that when she's aware you're watching porn she feels unimportant to you, or unattractive, or pushed away, don't disagree or even reassure her. Start by trying to understand how she feels, and why; when you do, let her know it—not by saying so, but by paraphrasing what she's telling you. Without correcting it or judging it.

This is no small thing. When your partner feels understood it's easier to have a rational conversation about the options you have as a couple.

But what about her concerns? Year by year she gets older and, um, rounder—and the actresses you watch stay young and firm. She has the sense that you're enjoying the heck out of something to which she's not invited—which isn't the way you two usually do things—right?. Even if she's not jealous of the actresses who entertain you, she knows that you're experiencing sexual highlights without her. She's not part of your fantasies (our regular partners seldom are), and she's not there when you have your moments of intense pleasure.

And she assumes this isn't temporary.

You're gone, enjoying a new hobby that you two don't discuss. For some women, it feels like there's a void in their own home. Like if you discovered she had a new friend whom you knew almost nothing about, and whom you two never discussed. And that you knew you probably never would.

And she's undoubtedly seen at least one story somewhere about how dangerous porn is for both users and their families. It probably seemed quite authoritative.

So how do you suppose she feels about all this?

I don't expect you to know. I expect you to wonder. That's curiosity.

I don't expect you to know. I expect you to suppose—it might be this, it might be that. I expect you to imagine how you'd feel if the positions were reversed. That's empathy.

This is how you get beyond the "porn is crap," *"no it's not,"* "porn demeans women," *"no it doesn't"* non-conversation: with curiosity and empathy. So your conversations about porn can get past the porn part—to the people and to their relationship. To you and her.

Interlude G

IS THERE SUCH A THING AS GAY (OR STRAIGHT) PORN?

We know there's porn and we know there are gay people. But is there "gay porn?" Or is it simply porn featuring people of the same gender having sex together?

If it's "gay porn," then we would be surprised to find straight people looking at it. If it's porn featuring same-gender sex, however, then we'd be surprised if there *weren't* straight people watching it.

It's the latter, of course. Adults find all sorts of fantasies and images sexy—and they don't necessarily have anything to do with their real-life desires. That is, enjoying scenes of two men having oral sex doesn't make a man gay. Similarly, enjoying looking at fictional scenes of sexual coercion (or fantasizing being raped) doesn't mean a person wants that in real life.

To put it another way, what arouses us is only part of our sexual orientation. If you want to know if someone's gay, straight, or bi, ask them who they have sex with (and who they want to have sex with in real life), not what videos they like to watch.

The question came up in a professional conversation the other day, when an inexperienced therapist asked why some straight men were attracted to websites featuring pre-operative transsexuals (typically advertised as "tranny," "she-male," or "lady-boy" porn)—that is, images of people with women's breasts and a penis.

Why wouldn't they? Talk about having your cake and eating it too! Most straight men enjoy women's breasts, and most straight men are fascinated with penises. This porn allows the viewer to enjoy both at the same time. And the arithmetical possibilities—whether the performer is onscreen with one other person or several—are increased geometrically. A fellatio train, anyone? Domination-submission-domination-submission, anyone?

That's why I discourage my straight patients from using the expression "gay fantasy," and discourage my gay patients from saying "straight fantasy" (unless they're fantasies *about* being gay or straight, which is a different matter). These expressions actually cloud things, because they suggest that the enjoyment of cross-orientation fantasies needs explanation.

An investigation can be valuable, of course, especially if people have trouble thinking about or acknowledging their interests or curiosity. Sometimes the content of a favorite fantasy is a metaphor or an indirect expression of interest. A same-gender fantasy may excite a straight person because of, say, power dynamics. A mixed-gender fantasy may excite a gay person because of, say, a sense of belonging.

It turns out that sexuality is more complicated than gay-or-straight. In 1948, Alfred Kinsey presented data showing that "the world is not simply divided into sheep and goats," and presented his 7-point Kinsey Scale of sexual orientation. These days, expressions like GLBTQQ remind us that a person's sexual orientation is a movie, not a photograph; interests, aspirations, and behavior can change over time. Curiosity and experimentation can take us in unexpected (sometimes even boring) directions. In that sense, we're all "queer," and potentially or actually "questioning."

Ultimately, it's more important to enjoy our fantasies than to understand or decode them. Most of us enjoy mainstream entertainment—whether violent video games, syrupy romance novels, detailed historical documentaries, or utopian science fiction films—without wondering what our preferences for these things "mean." We all know perfectly gentle people who enjoy the brutal weekly mayhem on *CSI* or *Bones* or whatever the latest adrenalin-pumper is. We may criticize their taste, but we don't need to fear their violent impulses.

Unless, of course, we try to change the channel.

Interlude H

HOW TO WATCH A LOT OF PORN AND HAVE GOOD PARTNER SEX, TOO

Say you watch a lot of porn.

Say you want to have really enjoyable sex.

Some people say you have to choose one or the other.

Some say that porn changes your brain so you can't enjoy sex with a real person. Nonsense. If you don't want sex with a real person, it's either because you don't desire the person you're with, or because you have issues about sex or closeness. That's when watching porn is a lot easier than creating good sex. But let's not blame the porn.

Some say that porn gives you unrealistic ideas about sex. Yes, that happens—unrealistic ideas about what people look like, sound like, do, want, and about how communication and hugging have very little place in sex. Unrealistic ideas about sex—whether you get them from porn, from religion, from *Cosmopolitan*, or from your father—make it hard to create enjoyable sex.

And some say that porn provides such powerful images that we inevitably compare our own sex to the images—and of course we seem pretty lame in comparison. Yes, that happens. That even happens to people who don't look at porn, who have sex with someone who does. They imagine you're thinking about porn when you make love, which makes them think about porn when they make love, and that's bad for sex all the way around.

Some people say the solution is to stop watching porn. Probably not gonna happen. And probably wouldn't solve most of the problem anyway.

Rather, I say the solution is to make love consciously, and to watch porn consciously. That helps to keep the two activities separate, which is the key to enjoying both.

So if you want to watch a lot of porn *and* have good sex, here's what to do:

- Remember that porn is fiction. It's not a documentary, it's a highlight reel. It involves lighting, editing, and off-camera preparation. It's planned ahead of time so that everything looks perfect.
- During partner sex, learn how to focus your attention on your body—how your partner's hair smells, how your partner's nipple tastes, how your partner's skin feels, and so on. Center your sexual experience in what you're *feeling* rather than in what you're thinking.
- Don't expect sex to feel how porn looks. That's like expecting driving your car to feel like driving a Maserati looks. Or expecting playing tennis to feel like Wimbledon looks. Reality can't compete with created images. We have to value reality for itself.
- Know what your partner likes and wants. That won't match what people do in porn films. Adjust your expectations accordingly.
- Budget plenty of time to explore your partner's desires, and find the ones that you enjoy.
- Remember that unlike watching a porn film, orgasm isn't the point. The goal of sex is to enjoy yourself and to feel glad you're alive. Orgasm lasts maybe five seconds. Do the math—five seconds out of 20 minutes of sex isn't much. Learn to enjoy the rest of the sex. Learn to create sex that you enjoy.
- Be flexible if things don't go exactly as you want. You can be ashamed, angry, or afraid, or you can move closer to your partner, gently smile, and say, "Well, let's go ahead and do something else, right?"
- In general, talk more and screw less. You'll get more out of the experience, and you're more likely to get more chances. Kiss more and screw less. Caress more and screw less. Laugh more and screw less. Whisper more and screw less. Sex—and whispering and kissing—is for people. Porn is for paid professionals. Make love, not porn.
- Ask a friendly question every time you have sex: Do you like this? Would you like that better if I went faster? Is that a good "Oh!" or a problem "Oh!"? People don't do that on camera—which is part of what can make real sex better than porn.

So sure, you can watch a lot of porn and enjoy sex with a real person. You just have to remember which is which.

Interlude I

DOES PORN DEMEAN WOMEN?

I don't think this is a very helpful question.

Porn is a compendium of human fantasies about sexuality—and, therefore, about power, pleasure, connection, anger, fear, gender, desire, beauty, comfort, the exotic, and many other things.

Of course, human sexuality involves enormous doses of imagination. That's part of what gives it so much impact in our lives.

So when some people criticize that "porn demeans women," I wonder if they're objecting to men's and women's sexual imaginations, or men's and women's sexual behavior, or to some hypothesized interaction between the two.

A small amount of porn depicts male characters committing violent acts against female characters who seem to be suffering. Watching this appears to be erotic for some men (and more than a few women). Some people don't like this fact—a fact that shouldn't be blamed on porn. Do these depictions "demean women?" No. They are fictional portrayals that many people find distasteful, which is a quite different thing. They show situations, emotions, behaviors—and yes, sometimes cruelty—drawn from the human sexual imagination.

This material represents a very small amount of pornography, precisely because most consumers do not find such things erotically engaging—which is the whole point of watching porn.

On the other hand, some amount of porn depicts characters engaged in erotic power play: teasing, spanking, constraining, controlling, pretend coercion. Men and women have found stories, music, or pictures of such things exciting throughout history. And many lovers do these or related activities in real life. In the world of human sexuality, power is a primary currency, so our sexual imagination is rich with it.

This power dynamic in consenting relationships is paradoxical: two people cooperatively agree to divide up power in an asymmetrical way for a specified time period (the asymmetrical arrangement typically ends when the sex is finished, sometimes even sooner). For erotic purposes, they then pretend this division of power is real and not under their control. So regardless of handcuffs or stern words or candle wax, this dynamic really exists only in the imagination. Depicting this visually is an artistic challenge, whether for pornography or Sharon Stone, for Andy Warhol or Jane Campion.

So does porn demean women?

Aside from the overt violence (*not* the pretend coercion of sexual games common in both porn and real-life sex) of interest to a very small number of consumers, what else does porn typically depict that some people critique as demeaning to women?

Fictional depictions of female lust. Female sexual desire. Female exhibitionism. Female submission. Female domination. Women flaunting their bodies. Woman–woman sex. Women taking joy in their sexual pleasure. Women taking joy in their partner's pleasure. Women wanting whatever mental or physical satisfaction that sex seems to be offering in a given situation.

Why would anyone object to any of these fictional depictions? If those things are demeaning to women, how wholesome, how puerile, how stripped of eroticism does a woman's sexuality need to be before victim-oriented "feminists" like John Stoltenberg, Rebecca Whisnant, or Catharine MacKinnon say it is not "demeaning" to her?

* * *

To say that porn demeans women is to deny the reality of some women's passion, lust, and desire. It's to say that women never enjoy what men enjoy. It's to say that women don't enjoy playing games with their sexuality, including power games. It's to say that women shouldn't be who they are or enjoy who they are, but that they can only enjoy "authentic" sexuality within limited (and historically stereotypical) bounds.

This is *not* feminism.

Saying that men are exploiting women when men are enjoying female eroticism is what demeans women. It objectifies women and cheapens the eroticism they create. To say that women are being exploited when a male gaze is enjoying their pleasure or enjoying images of female eroticism is to rip the partners' collaboration out of sex. It actually says that female sexuality is defined by the male gaze, that the male gaze trivializes female eroticism. No, female eroticism has its own authenticity and integrity whether men are observing or not—meaning yes, it has authenticity even when men *are* observing.

Exactly what version of (1) female sexuality and of (2) male-female erotic interaction is being promoted by pathologizing female passion, and the male enjoyment of it?

Does this mean a woman can't dress sexy for her lover? Can't dance for her lover? That a woman can't give her body to her lover? Does it mean that women have to control their eroticism lest it excite men too much? Does it mean men and women can't play power games in bed? That they can't use sex to pretend they are different creatures than they actually are?

If—*if*—in the act of watching a porn film a man reduces the actress to a body, to an object, why is this bad? If it is, why then is it OK to watch Meryl Streep, with her fake accents, wig, and scripted lines, who is merely a vessel for the ideas of the playwright and director? And why then is it OK to watch professional athletes, dancers, and singers, who indeed sacrifice their health and comfort to train and then perform for us? If the answer is, "Because our objectification of athletes and other performers takes place within a specific space," the same is true for pornography.

Do we care about the person inside of LeBron James, Serena Williams, Miley Cyrus, or other celebrities? Do we really care when a rich football star says his abused body won't let him get on the floor to play with his kids, or that a young television celebrity makes a series of bad life choices? For that matter, do I care about my letter carrier as a person, or do I only care that he does his job, no matter how much his feet hurt or his back's been injured?

The issue of relating to people merely as impersonal entities performing a task is a fundamental critique of capitalism, and it's worth a discussion. But porn didn't invent this problem. And if this dynamic seems "worse" because sex is involved, that reflects our attitude about sexuality rather than a sophisticated analysis. It does *not* represent some special kind of compassion for people who perform in adult films—who, by the way, aren't asking for anyone's special compassion. They want what the cashiers at Walmart want—a raise, better health insurance, and the flexibility to leave work early when their kid gets sick.

If men get inaccurate ideas about women from porn, does it mean that porn demeans women? Virtually all media products involve exaggerated ideas about human beings—from Euripides' *Medea* 2,500 years ago to the Bronte sisters, *The Merchant of Venice*, Sherlock Holmes, the Supremes, and John Wayne, for starters. The National Football League provides inaccurate ideas about men every Sunday. Do we stop watching movies, professional sports, video games, Broadway productions? Do we stop listening to music, stop looking at paintings? No. To best enrich our lives by consuming the creations of imaginary worlds by artists or performers we value, we simply need a bit of media literacy—not to stop watching or listening.

Although a small amount of pornography depicts gruesome behavior, not only does porn not demean women, most of it celebrates female sexuality—typically without the culturally redemptive context of love, relationship, intimacy, etc. This is what people from across the political spectrum find so upsetting. Demeaning to women—that women are imagined as truly sexual beings? Really?

Interlude J

45 HELPFUL THINGS YOU CAN LEARN FROM PORN

Pornography is not meant to be educational. It's fiction, period.

Nevertheless, given the abstinence-oriented sex "education" most young people get, most families' and couples' discomfort discussing sex seriously, and Christianity's taboos about sexual reality, most people need more information about sexuality.

If they're fortunate, they manage to find a smart book or two, a reliable website or two, a grownup with some accurate information, and maybe even an enlightened, open-minded, communicative sex partner. Anyone lacking all four who wants sex information almost inevitably turns to porn, whether intentionally or not.

Unfortunately, many young people don't realize that porn is not a documentary. Lacking porn literacy and media literacy, they're ignorant about editing, off-camera preparation, and other normal features of filmmaking. People who lack real-world sexual experience may have trouble understanding some of the complex things they see in porn, like depictions of BDSM.

While some people assume that sex is—or should be—like what they see in porn, every good sex educator cautions against this (I certainly have, over and over). That said, let's not forget the helpful things consumers can learn from porn.

This is *not, not, not* to say that everything people learn from porn is good. Puh-leeze—any 17-year-old who thinks his next girlfriend is dying for anal sex or a chance to go down on the pizza delivery guy is in for a shock. And it's always too bad when men think most women climax from 90 seconds of intercourse (although the antidote is pretty straightforward: a woman simply telling a guy "that's not me," with no apology necessary).

So here's a reminder of helpful things that porn can teach us about sex.

Wait, one more time: I know, I know—porn also contains many inaccurate, even egregious lessons. But if we're concerned about people taking those wrong lessons seriously, let's also take these potentially helpful lessons seriously. Sex educators have been teaching many of them for years, and we should be glad to have them reinforced.

45 Helpful Things You Can Learn from Porn

Men can touch their penises during sex
Women can touch their vulvas during sex
Spit works for lube
Some women sometimes desire sex without romance
Telling each other stories can make sex hotter
Men can climax using their own hand
Some people like to look at each other during sex
Some women think about sex in advance
Women sometimes use their hand to insert the penis into their vagina
Men sometimes use their hand to insert their penis into a vagina
If the penis comes out during intercourse, you can simply put it back in
Some women like fellatio
Some women like cunnilingus
Some men like fellatio
Some men like cunnilingus
Some people enjoy having the outside of their anus licked
Some people enjoy licking their partner's anus
Men and women can enjoy intercourse with a condom
People can kiss during sex
Different people kiss really differently
Even women who enjoy intercourse may like their clitoris stimulated
People can change position during sex
Vulvas can look really different from each other
There's more to a vulva than just a vagina
Some women use and enjoy vibrators and dildos
Some men like their balls stimulated during sex
Watching someone undress can be sexy
Pregnant women can be sexual
Whether during intercourse, oral, or manual sex, the clitoris can be important
The volume of ejaculate is not related to penis size
Sex is more than penis–vagina intercourse
Some women have orgasms

Some people are on very friendly terms with ejaculate
Some older women and older men are sexual
Older women can be attractive to younger men (and vice versa)
People can have sex with people of different races
Heterosexual people can enjoy watching same-gender sex
Women with small breasts can enjoy having their breasts stimulated
Some people enjoy hair-pulling, spanking, and teasing as part of sex
People can smile and talk to each other during sex
People can indicate to each other what they like during sex
Some women shave/wax their vulvas, others don't
Some men shave/wax their pubic area, others don't
A man can happily ejaculate outside a vagina
People don't have to climax at the same time for sex to be great

Whatever your sexual fantasy, you're not the only one who has it.

PART III

About You and Yours

Chapter Four

YOUR KIDS AND PORN

First, the good news: your kids are safer than you probably fear.

Porn is not a toxic substance that can infect them. Porn doesn't make them run out and molest other kids. Porn doesn't make them want to rape or get raped. Porn won't make them a porn addict, even if they worry that they're a porn addict. And if they sleep in and miss school, porn didn't make them do it (the culprit is more likely Facebook or texting, although the kid is ultimately responsible).

Does that mean you shouldn't be concerned? No. But rather than succumbing to PornPanic and its phony, irrational dangers, here's what you might want to be concerned about regarding your kids and porn:

- Kids getting inaccurate ideas about sex; everyone seems to agree that this is a problem
- Kids confused about what they see
- Kids feeling guilty or ashamed of their sexual fantasies, thoughts, or feelings
- Kids feeling guilty or ashamed of the fact that they masturbate

The worst part of any of this is if they feel they can't talk with you about it. That is, the worst part of kids looking at porn is if they have visual or emotional experiences around sexuality that they can't discuss with you.

Yes, the strongest impact of kids' relationship with porn (as with many other things) involves the extent to which they're hiding from you, fearing you, learning from you, or being comforted by you. The problem, of course, is that porn is about sex, and most kids know you don't want them watching it. So without your special effort, they'll be highly disposed toward secrecy and isolation. That makes your feelings part of the situation you and your kids are facing regarding porn. Which, by the way, is one unspoken reason that some parents resent porn—"I don't want to talk about sex stuff with my kid, but porn forces me to."

So let's start with that.

Porn is an adult product, made for adult consumers. Kids can't really understand it. So they need guidance. If you wish, go ahead and tell your kids you don't want them watching it, and explain why—it's an adult product, made for adult consumers. There are things in it that will probably confuse them, maybe even trouble them. So tell them you strongly prefer they not watch until they're older.

Some kids will abide by your request. Others won't.

Now it's tricky for a parent to say, "I don't want you doing x, but if you do, here's how I want you to do it." But we do that with other things:

- "I don't want you drinking alcohol, but if you do, call me and I'll come and take you home."
- "I don't want you texting while you bike, but if you do, wear a helmet."
- "I don't want you having intercourse, but if you do, use contraception."
- "I don't want you in a car driven by Joe, but if you do, wear a seatbelt. And check that he hasn't been drinking."

So now you have to say that about porn, and that's where your familiar parenting values come in: "I don't want you watching porn, but if you do,

- I still love you.
- I still want you happy and healthy.
- I still want to help you understand your world and the world around you.
- I still want you to understand that both sexuality and relationships can be great or not so great, depending on how you manage them.
- I still want you to feel we can talk about anything.
- I still want to teach you how to make good choices about sexuality and relationships.

If you observe that none of these are specifically about porn, you're absolutely right. The most important rule about parenting kids around the issue of porn is . . . don't get distracted by the porn.

So let's say you're a good parent, and you know the routine on "I don't want you doing x, but let's discuss how to do it more safely." But what about *this* x?

That's a fair question, and a helpful answer requires some context. We've discussed how America's PornPanic affects us in many ways; so how does it affect parenting? By scaring us into believing that (1) our kids are in great danger from watching porn; (2) our kids are in great danger from others watching porn; (3) talking to kids about porn in a reasonable way will harm them, harm our relationship with them, and/or harm our kid's relationship to others.

That urging you to believe your only reasonable option is mobilizing to keep them from watching it, and that other than "keep away," there's nothing about which to educate them. That if you're not frightened or angry about porn's effects on your kids, you're a bad parent.

Of course, a certain amount of the dangerism surrounding kids and porn involves sexuality in general. For example, many activists warn that viewing porn leads young people to premarital sex, masturbation, and believing that recreational sex is acceptable. Now some parents find that prospect way less frightening than others (you may be wondering, "And the problem with that is . . . ?"). But when sex-negative messages are mixed with porn-negative messages (e.g., "Porn teaches male viewers to hate women"), the combination can look frightening to even the most open-minded parent.

Here are some common allegations about how porn harms kids. They are repeated so frequently and loudly that many people assume they're actual facts—but they're not. According to anti-porn activists:

- Porn ruins kids for future relationships
- Porn trains their brains (badly)
- Porn lowers their current and later adult opinion of women
- Porn leads them to molest other children
- Porn addicts them
- Porn sexualizes them too early
- Porn sets them up for erection or other sex problems in early adulthood

These supposed outcomes lend an air of urgency and pessimism to the project of keeping kids away from porn. It's no surprise that so many parents give up before they start.

If you feel frightened or powerless, remember: This dangerist narrative is being driven by people who don't care about your family, but do have a vested interest in your insecurity. And do remember that just as parents are the primary sex educators of their children, they're the primary porn educators of their children. To do that properly, it's important that you know the facts about these **common myths.**

- *Myth:* Porn Ruins Kids for Future Sexual Relationships

While porn does present images of sexuality that don't reflect real life, so do many other popular media. Parents can compensate for that by discussing actual sexuality (you know, beyond plumbing) with young people. It's sexual ignorance, not sexual imagery, that can damage future sexual relationships.

- *Myth:* Porn Trains Their Brains (Badly)

There's no evidence for sporadic porn viewing ruining anyone's brain. Our brains are always changing, and our brain responds to pleasure in all its forms: playing with a puppy (even watching videos of people playing with a puppy), eating a cookie, seeing parents smile, listening to a favorite song, and watching pictures of naked people having sex.

Very few young people watch porn frequently and intensely enough to fall into a different category. Of course the satisfaction of watching porn reinforces interest in watching it again. Most young people have competing interests—sports, school, video games, friends, social media. Every good parent encourages these interests (other than social media), irrespective of porn.

- *Myth:* Porn Lowers Their Opinions of Women

There's no evidence for this.

Teach kids to respect women by respecting women—at home, on the street, and in the news. If you have daughters, talk to them about the various ways you perceive them using their looks or sexuality. At the same time, teach them that their sexuality is a valuable part of them, not something to be denigrated by anyone.

If you have sons, make it clear that women are, first and foremost, people. Then teach them, day after day, how to treat people. If your son has an older sister, encourage him to ask her questions about how guys behave with her—especially the ways she doesn't like. Invite him to think about how he wants people treating her, and to compare that with his own treatment of the girls in his life. And let him know that women who enjoy sex are to be valued, not judged.

- *Myth:* Porn Leads Kids to Molest Other Children

There's no evidence for this.

Teach kids to respect other children—at home, on the street, and in the news. This includes diversity, gender, anger control, self-soothing, empathy, and non-violence.

Forcing other kids to kiss you, or touch you, or let you touch them is wrong, but not because it involves sex; it's wrong to force other kids to do stuff, period.

And by the way, kids have been playing doctor since before there were doctors. It's absolutely natural for kids to be curious about each other's bodies and their own erotic feelings. Don't confuse cooperative kid play with "molestation" just because there's eroticism or genitalia involved.

- *Myth:* Porn Addicts Them

There's no such thing as "porn addiction." And while the satisfaction of watching porn reinforces interest in watching it again, that's also true of kids' other activities, like sports, friends, social media, and family. So definitely encourage their interest in activities and relationships you think are healthy.

In general, kids need limits placed on their screen time, regardless of what's on the screen. We should be way more concerned about kids becoming "addicted" to texting and screen time in general than to their possible porn "addiction."

- *Myth:* Porn Sexualizes Kids Too Early

What exactly does this mean? Our culture has become more sexually oriented since the Internet came to most homes 20 years ago. These days, you can buy vibrators online; TV includes nudity and coarse language; popular music is filled with sexual references that are far beyond the old Moon-June-Spoon days; and the news media discuss sexual issues like Viagra, abortion, sex work, campus rape, transgenderism, and sexting in ways unthinkable just a few years ago.

As our culture evolves, we need to adjust our parenting accordingly. Singling out porn as the vehicle that (negatively) sexualizes them is unhelpful. Instead, we should be talking to kids about the sexualization of their everyday experience: What do you think of girls who dress that way? When you feel pressured to sext, what do you do? Ever have a sexual feeling you felt embarrassed about? Do you feel you need to compete with other, cooler kids using your sexuality? What do you think of the lyrics to your favorite songs?

Over and over, I observe that people moaning the loudest about kids getting sexualized too early are the most uncomfortable that kids are sexual beings. Regardless of how exploitative our culture is, our kids' sexuality is a healthy part of them. It's our job to give them tools to navigate a world that's overly focused on sex.

- *Myth:* Porn Sets Kids Up for Erection or Other Sex Problems in Early Adulthood

There's no evidence for this. Erection and other sex problems can result from a wide variety of sources, including endocrine, medication side effects, neurological issues, and emotional issues like guilt, shame, and isolation. The way to best ensure your child's healthy adult sex life is by talking about sex honestly, making it clear that diversity is the hallmark of human sexual imagination and preference, and letting your child know you're available to respond to all questions about sex.

* * *

So as you consider what's *not* a problem, consider what is. Here's what you should be concerned about regarding your kids watching porn:

- Kids Can Get Inaccurate Ideas About What Sex Is Like in Real Life

Everyone agrees that kids (and adults, for that matter) get inaccurate ideas about sex from looking at porn. But people disagree on how to respond. The best solution is to talk about sex as it is—not to condemn porn, hide sex, or shame kids, but to explain what they're dealing with and to counter some of its challenges.

It's impossible to discuss porn's inaccuracies, conventions, and limitations without talking about sex accurately. That, of course, includes issues like why people have sex; what it's like; the difference (or connection) between what the bodies do and how the people feel; how people decide when and with whom to be sexual; and the common consequences of poor sexual decision-making. Adults spend a lifetime figuring out answers to these questions; so you're all ready to discuss these with your kid, right?

Just like kids need media literacy so they can use TV, video games, blogs, and popular music in healthy ways, kids need porn literacy (despite the fact that you'd rather they not watch porn). They need to understand that they're watching actors playing roles and following scripts, not real couples in documentaries. They need to understand that just as *Glee* and *Harry Potter* are scripted and edited, so are porn films—and that most of what the actors do is determined by camera angles and lighting, not by their personal preferences. None of these media products is an accurate portrayal of real life.

Porn usually omits crucial parts of sex:

~ the feelings
~ the kissing
~ the caressing and embracing

~ the laughing
~ the talking

Together, these create the connecting, which most adults say is an important part of sex much of the time.

Here are some other ways that porn sex is different than real-life sex. In real life:

~ Most people don't look like that (perfect breasts, butts, faces, and genitalia)
~ Most men don't get or stay erect so easily
~ Most couples need lubricant for genital insertion
~ Most people don't usually do many commonly shown things (including anal sex, threesomes, sex with strangers, intercourse without birth control, ejaculating on someone's face)
~ While sex can be wonderful, most of the time it isn't an incredibly intense experience
~ Most people don't have sex in public or in physically awkward places or positions

In short, sex in real life usually doesn't look like, sound like, or feel like sex in porn looks like, sounds like, or appears to feel like.

• Kids Can Get Confused About What They See

Any reasonable kid watching porn would have lots of questions: Is that what sex is really like? Is that what most people look like naked? Do strangers really have sex together so easily? Why do people switch from smiling to moaning or screaming so abruptly? And what are they moaning or screaming about? Do most girls like to kiss girls? Are some people really rough with each other in bed—and doesn't it hurt?

Those are actually some of the most common questions that kids ask sex education websites.

Any normal kid would be confused seeing a half-hour of even the most mundane real-life lovemaking, because it involves things so far outside of their experience. Most adults take most aspects of sex for granted: the pacing, the nudity, the various changes of position and activity, the way the bodies do or don't fit together, the interruptions (bathroom break, leg cramp, lost erection, need for rest, etc.), the increasing (or intermittent) arousal, the smiling, the anxiety, the orgasm, the sense (or lack) of connection, the pursuit of mutual pleasure. If you've never had sex, or have only had a hurried, anxious, or drunk experience, the whole thing would be baffling to observe.

As real people continue experimenting with BDSM, sex toys, and other kinds of games, porn increasingly features these things as well. Viewing such scenes would be confusing to any kid.

To address that, you can explain that just as kids play games on the ballfield, pretending to be mean or brave when they really aren't, some adults play games in bed, pretending to be bossy or submissive when they really aren't.

And when people play rough sex games—"which of course you can't understand right now because you have so little experience with all of this"—they have limits about exactly how rough they want to get. No one likes to really get hurt—you'll notice that no one is punching anyone, no one is bleeding, and no one is stopping things, even though they could. And remember, the really, really rough stuff is play-acting, with actors and actresses following movie scripts they've approved in advance—like pro wrestling on TV or bar fights in movie westerns.

What if your kid asks why people watch this stuff in the first place? That's actually a great question. In general, adults watch porn because they feel it makes masturbating more exciting and enjoyable. It may remind them of what they've done and enjoyed, or it's exotic and they imagine enjoying it, or they don't want to do it, but they like watching other people do it—like wrestling with sharks or drag racing. Yes, many adults periodically like to get themselves sexually excited. They generally masturbate while watching; if they watch with their partner, it's usually before or during sex.

And why do people watch BDSM stuff in particular? It's because some adults find games of dominance and submission exciting—either to do or to watch. "If you find that confusing, well, that's OK—porn is for adults, remember?" If you like, you can even mention that many adults (both those who do it and those who don't) find BDSM confusing as well.

- Kids Can Feel Guilty or Ashamed of Their Sexual Fantasies, Thoughts, or Feelings

Almost all young people have sexual thoughts or feelings, and many kids feel uncomfortable, even horrified, by theirs. Generally, no one else in the family talks about their sexual fantasies, thoughts, or feelings; and their friends aren't likely to talk about fantasizing about a sibling, much-older neighbor, much-younger cousin, etc. So they might feel isolated and unable to process the intensity of the feeling or the fear that they're abnormal. Most adults know that the rules of fantasy and of real life can be contradictory; kids are still learning to separate the two, which can make the realm of sexuality even more confusing.

Watching porn encourages sexual fantasizing. And it can launch kids in new and different directions of erotic thought and feeling, which are simply too unfamiliar or intense to process properly. And porn can lead to kids looking at familiar people in brand new ways; for example, watching an actress close to Mother's age who acts very sexual may lead a kid to think of Mother as sexual for the first time. Finally, watching porn can invite a kid to fantasize more frequently, making situational factors (like a cousin sleeping over the house) a springboard for new fantasies, whether one-time or ongoing.

- Kids Can Feel Guilty or Ashamed of the Fact That They Masturbate

You are OK about your kid masturbating, right? Well, more or less OK? That's a key point here; if you aren't, the whole conversation about porn is moot, because that's most of the point of looking at porn. Perhaps your kid isn't yet masturbating per se (stroking his/her genitalia to arousal and usually climax), but is just deliberately becoming aroused by squirming, muscle movements, or rubbing against an object such as a teddy bear; for many parents disturbed by masturbation per se, that's often equally distressing.

Kids don't ask our permission to start masturbating (and you wouldn't exactly want that, right?), and whether we're aware of it or not, they generally start earlier than we think is reasonable ("Only 26, and starting to masturbate, Brian? Oh, they grow up so quickly."). As with every part of child development, different kids discover themselves sexually at very different ages; and as with every part of their development, they need to know that they're OK, and not dramatically different from other, presumably "normal," kids.

In western culture, feeling guilty about masturbation has been common for centuries.

Many otherwise-sophisticated American adults, in fact, are embarrassed that they do it, and many admonish their partners against doing it. Of course, such adults are likely to pass on this rejection of masturbation to their kids, intentionally or not.

During the Victorian era, masturbation was seen as a dangerous sign of moral weakness. Many people believed a non-meat diet would help curb masturbation, which is why clergymen Sylvester Graham and John Harvey Kellogg invented crackers and corn flakes respectively (yes, really). Some well-meaning parents forced their sons to wear spiked metal devices around their penises that would cause pain if a child became aroused. Many "progressive" parents tied their kids' wrists to their bedposts at night so they couldn't touch themselves while dreaming.

We're somewhat less barbaric about it now, but millions of parents—especially those who self-identify as born-again or evangelical Christian—warn their kids against the practice (if they talk about it at all) or freak out when they "catch" their kid doing it. Notice the common description—"catching" a kid touching himself, sounding the same way as if we'd "caught" a kid sneaking an extra cookie or tormenting the family dog.

Of course, there are advantages to masturbation. It gives young people a sense of ownership of their bodies, and it helps develop the sexual self-awareness that can make later partner sex more enjoyable. For adolescents with sexual urges, it's a form of sexual expression that doesn't risk pregnancy, infection, or heartbreak.

Once kids discover the pleasure of masturbating they're unlikely to stop, and once they experience how porn enhances masturbation, they're not likely to stop that, either. If you're going to tell a kid masturbation is wrong, you'll need some sort of reason that (1) acknowledges their sexual feelings and (2) won't undermine their future sexuality. I'm afraid I can't help you on this because I can't think of a single good reason kids shouldn't masturbate.

The only way a parent can really discourage a kid from masturbation is by scaring the hell out of him or by filling the kid with high levels of shame and guilt (although history proves that this usually fails to limit masturbation or any other sexual outlet). A parent considering this approach should be clear that that's their intention—to damage their kid psychologically—and possibly discuss this goal with the family doctor.

* * *

Clearly, it's much easier to discuss porn-related issues if a special parent–child relationship around sexuality already exists. That special relationship involves trust, openness, the ability to disagree lovingly, some vocabulary, and discussions about values and the diversity of the human family (including the fact that a parent and child might ultimately have different sexual ideas, goals, and experiences).

Regardless of your child's age, you don't want a discussion of pornography to be the first conversation you have about sex. So put this book down right now and begin a conversation with your child about sex that *doesn't* involve porn. You'll be preparing both of you for the porn-oriented conversations that are surely coming—sooner than (either of) you might prefer.

Similarly, you don't want your first parent–child discussion about porn to involve conflict or punishment—so start a conversation with your kid about this as soon as you can. Don't wait until you feel entirely comfortable!

PORN LITERACY CHECKLIST FOR KIDS

(Parents, feel free to hand this to your kid, read this to your kid, or share this with your kid. And feel free to use it yourself. It applies to all people consuming pornography.)

Like the fictional worlds of *Harry Potter, Star Trek,* and *Twilight,* pornography depicts a world that looks familiar but doesn't actually exist. It features bodies most people don't have, doing things most people don't do, in situations most people are never in.

It would be a big mistake to assume that you live in that world. Because sex in real life isn't like sex in porn. It can't be, because what we see is the product of acting and editing—not real relationships or real situations.

If you're going to watch porn, remember that your life can't be like the lives of the characters you see there. Real people—like you—generally don't have as much desire, get as excited, or feel so intensely as the characters in porn. That's because you're real, and the characters aren't.

Porn leaves out a lot of what most people enjoy about sex: kissing, hugging, whispering, laughing, and talking afterwards. Real sex often includes words of genuine affection, which porn almost never includes. That's because the characters in porn generally don't feel that close to each other.

Because porn is a complex product, consuming it without understanding it can be confusing. And because sexuality is an important part of life, getting confused about it while watching porn can cause anyone—especially young people—difficulty. So here's a list of what *everyone* watching porn of *any* kind needs to understand. Any item that you can't honestly check, think it over before watching again. If you just can't make sense of it, ask an adult you trust (yeah, I know, hard to just relax and talk about this with Mom, Dad, or Uncle Louis). If you don't know an adult you can ask personally, ask the cool folks at either www.Scarleteen.com or www.GoAskAlice.columbia.edu.

(continued)

PORN LITERACY CHECKLIST FOR KIDS (*continued*)

[ ] I know that porn is fiction, not real.

[ ] I know professional porn is shot with actors and actresses following a script, using special lighting and camera angles, and that the film is edited to create a finished product that looks like it really happened.

[ ] I know that actors and actresses prepare themselves off-camera right before a shoot with products like Viagra, enemas, and lubricants (not to mention yoga and back exercises) to help create the images I see.

[ ] I realize I know nothing about porn actors and actresses as people.

[ ] I understand that most people don't have bodies like porn performers.

[ ] I understand that some recurring images in porn (such as ejaculating on someone's face, anal sex, threesomes, sudden sex without talking and relating first) are theatrical devices and don't reflect what most women or men want in sex.

[ ] I understand that people are paid to act in porn films and wouldn't do it for free.

[ ] I understand that most people aren't as uninhibited as the characters portrayed by porn performers.

[ ] I understand that most women don't want rough play or violence in their sex.

[ ] I understand that demonstrations of dominance and submission are cooperatively staged and end the second the camera is turned off.

[ ] I understand that a lot of the arousal and orgasm I see in porn is pretend, not real.

[ ] I understand that porn is made by adults for adults. If I don't understand the many good reasons minors should not watch porn, I should ask an adult I trust.

Chapter Five

SEXTING: WHO DOES IT?
HOW DOES IT AFFECT KIDS?

Your teen's phone has more computer power than the combined Allied Forces had when they defeated Hitler in 1945. It has more computer power than all of NASA had in 1969 when it sent two astronauts to the moon.[1]

And according to Moore's Law, in the time between me writing this and you reading it, your teen's computing power will almost certainly increase.[2]

So we give teens the most sophisticated and powerful communications device in the history of the world—and then get upset when they use it. Especially when they use it with all the limited wisdom a teenage brain can muster: texting while they bike, playing video games while they eat, Facebooking one friend while sitting with another. It's as if we've given all our kids bikes, neglect to teach them about traffic, rain, and how to keep their tires properly inflated, and then we're surprised and angry when they get into bike accidents.

And sexting: sending and/or receiving nude or sexually oriented photos of themselves or others. Most adults don't like that. In fact, adults have passed laws which throw teens in jail for sexting. That's some pretty serious disapproval.

So what's going on with sexting?

Some studies say at least one-quarter of kids do it[3]; other studies suggest only one in 25 do it.[4] The most popular sexts are photos of girls who are topless or naked, and of boys' penises. Why do they do it? David Finkelhor, director of the Crimes Against Children Research Center at the University of New Hampshire, says that kids do it as part of "risk taking" and "independence testing," pretty normal adolescent tasks.[5] In addition, kids sext for the same reasons that adults do various sexual activities: to express affection, to feel powerful, to gain prestige or popularity, to influence a partner or potential partner, to experience another's compliance, to satisfy curiosity, or to violate taboos.

Some parents fear that sexting means a kid is also having "real" sex. For better or worse, this isn't necessarily true. Because kids live online, sexting can be a form of sexual expression that's complete on its own. It can be a form of flirtation, or of what adults used to call "first base" (or "second base," or "third base," depending on who's keeping score). It can also be a silly form of just fooling around. And while it can be a way of getting attention, that doesn't mean it's pathological. And it doesn't mean that someone wants, or is about to, have "real" sex.

Like adults, young people have always used sexuality this way. If you conceptualize sexting as a normal sexual act within teen culture, it doesn't seem so unreasonable. With today's technology, however, it's now going on virtually and asynchronously (and perhaps less apologetically), and so society is trying to figure out what to do about it.

Adult feelings about teen sexting are complicated, because it sits at the intersection of two fundamental American anxieties: technology and adolescent sexuality. Teens today are doing what teens do—taking risks, experimenting, driving parents crazy. We've given them new tools with which to do this, and then we complain when they do. We're illiterate with those tools, making them scarier. And we won't talk to kids about it, except to say "don't do it."

Predictably, we're living through a society-wide panic about sexting. And so although it's legal in three-fourths of American states for 17-year-olds to have sex with each other, it's illegal for them to take or own photos of themselves or each other naked.[6] It's extremely difficult to explain that to an adolescent. It's impossible, of course, for the millions of parents who don't talk with their teens about sex at all.

In social welfare organizations, religious institutions, the media, and almost everywhere else, the topic of sexting immediately brings up questions of deviance, irresponsibility, and potential disaster. Implicit in this discourse are the ideas that sexuality is bad; that all sexual expression is morally equivalent and equally decadent; and that teen girls' sexuality is hazardous, requiring ongoing monitoring and control.

There's an interesting parallel between many activists denying that adult porn actresses could actually like performing in films, and many activists (often the same ones) denying that teen girls could actually like creating and sharing sexual images of themselves. Similarly, some activists think that sexual images of females—whether adults in pornography or teens who sext—are inherently dangerous, inviting violence, lowering the cultural status of women, and creating pressure on all women to behave more sexually than they wish. There seems to be little consciousness among these activists that adult women or teen women might want agency over their own sexuality, or that they shouldn't have to be responsible for patrolling the sexual behavior and relationships of others.

Some people anxiously predict that anyone with nude photos of themselves out in the world is just a mouse-click away from a ruined life.

But as digital natives, most teens understand something that most adults don't—that the way we live online has permanently changed our concepts (and the reality) of "privacy." And while no one knows exactly how this will turn out, we do know one thing: with as many as half of all teens sexting, and some percentage of those pictures leaking out beyond their intended audience, in 15 years a large number of dentists, high school teachers, journalists, social workers, pharmacists, venture capitalists, and everyone else will have nude pictures of themselves somewhere online.

It's similar to tattoos in the 1990s: Inked young people were warned they'd live disfigured and therefore marginalized forever. But 20 years later, it turns out that everyone's junior high school principal, gynecologist, grocery checker, and psychologist has one (or more) tattoos. Tats are here to stay, no longer considered a sign of pathology.

There are three possible problems with teen sexting. In increasing order of likelihood, they are:

1. Possibly adding to the supply of illegal child pornography online.
2. Compromising one's future with images that colleges, employers, and others might access and judge negatively.
3. Being charged with a crime, resulting in a jail sentence or even mandatory lifelong registration as a sex offender.

1. The first outcome is a problem in theory more than in practice. People who access illegal child porn frequently do so in a dark corner of the web that most people don't know exists and don't know how to find. Most child porn is traded among collectors in sophisticated networks that, again, are hard to find or join. Besides, people who want illegal child porn typically desire images of pre-pubescent children. And finally, there's no evidence that masses of people are trolling suburban email accounts or Facebook accounts trying to get a look at sexual images of local teens.

2. The second outcome is already changing, as Western society gets used to the reality that we all walk around with a camera every day, taking and then posting pictures of our mundane lives—sober and drunk, dressed up and dressed down, working hard and skipping work, and in varying states of provocative undress or flirtation.

The social disapproval that used to attach to erotic public behavior is almost gone as well. With actresses seamlessly moving from porn to mainstream films, and pop stars making nude music videos, and media icons wearing see-through dresses on Hollywood's red carpets, the social disapproval of nude selfies is declining as well. Whether with nude selfies, same-gender sexual play, polyamory, BDSM fashion, or queer identities requiring new personal pronouns, a whole generation is living with the slightly disdainful, nonchalant attitude of "What's the problem? It's only sex."

3. Being charged with a crime is far and away the most damaging outcome sexters are likely to incur. Ironically, it is the one that we as a society have the most power to change, yet are the least likely to address.

Contrary to popular fear, surveys consistently show that very few recipients of explicit selfies share them without the sender's consent. In fact, even pictures shared without consent generally travel between just two or three cellphones.[7] As with so many sensational sex-oriented urban legends, stories of sexting "rings" involving hundreds of students are the rare exception.

Regardless, the real issue with sexting is not the nudity or sexuality, it's consent: when images are either (1) created in malicious fashion the participant didn't authorize, or are (2) distributed in ways the creator has not authorized.

Amy Adele Hasinoff, Assistant Professor of Communication at the University of Colorado, says that our anxiety about technology and (teen girls') sexuality distract us from looking at the changing nature of privacy and consent. That's why our laws don't make distinctions between consensual sharing of and malicious distribution of private images. She challenges us to move beyond a simplistic understanding of female victimhood, seeing sexting as potentially an authentic expression of desire and agency.

This would refocus us on those who create or forward sexts without the subject's explicit consent.

While we would like for our teens to be wiser about creating (or allowing to be created) sexual images of themselves, forwarding these images is a big part of the problem—and is *not* solely the responsibility of the creator. If person A forwards a sext of person B without *explicit* permission, that's the person who should be criticized and shamed, rather than slut-shaming the person who's the subject of the image. This would require a change in both teen culture and adult culture. The sender might be criticized for poor judgment in trusting the wrong person, but that's hardly a flaw limited to teens.

As Hasinoff says, "Creating sexual images is not inherently harmful, but the malicious distribution of private images is."[8] Clementine Ford puts it even more strongly. She calls forwarding unauthorized texts stealing, and says that stolen sexts are a form of assault.[9]

So beyond the artificially created legal vulnerability, the only real problem around sexting is the non-consensual distribution of sexted images. This is *not* a good reason to ban sexting. Just as we don't tell people they can't own cars because their cars might be stolen, we shouldn't tell teens that they can't take or send nude selfies because the selfies might get stolen. Instead, we need to help kids understand how to sext more safely. While we're at it, we could even discuss alternatives to nude selfies (headless nude selfies? A new art form of "safe" nude photography?)—if we were willing to accept the legitimate impulses behind taking and sending them.

Figure 5.1 helps explain what's going on, and what should actually concern us.[10]

Starting on the left, "aggravated" sexting involves dynamics like coercion, deception, or even financial bribery. When adults are involved as either consumers or brokers, they are clearly violating the law—even if they are romantically involved with the sexter. Even when adults aren't involved, teens may be exploiting a would-be sexter either deliberately or through ignorance or naivete.

On the side called "experimental," teens may sext as an authentic expression of themselves, much as teens have done using other media in previous generations. Similarly, teens may sext because they feel pressured, want attention, want to prove something to themselves, want to defy authority, or want a thrill.

Clearly, the real problem is "aggravated" creation or distribution of sexts, not "experimental." But most states' school systems and legal system do recognize the difference.

Figure 5.1
Typologies of Youth-Produced Sexting Images

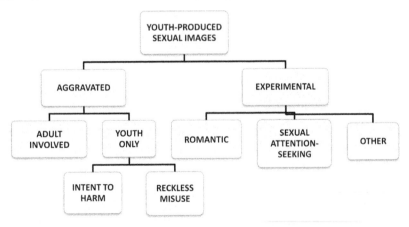

Source: Janis Wolak and David Finkelhor, Crimes Against Children Research Center, 2011.

Thus, in a world that facilitates sexting, with peer pressure to participate as creator, receiver, or forwarder, here's what we should be discussing with our kids:

- The idea that when anyone sends a sext *of themselves,* the recipient should assume that it is meant for them only and that they aren't authorized to forward it to *anyone;*
- The serious moral breakdown involved in forwarding a private text meant only for you, or consuming or forwarding a sext that wasn't meant for you;
- All the good reasons you shouldn't participate in non-consenting activity;
- Consent—how to ask for it, what it looks like, and what violations of consent look like;
- Various levels of trust, and how to know if/when you can trust someone, and in what domains.

Finally, because consent is a key aspect of the sexting issue, we need to discuss today's sexual double standard, which kids have absorbed from the adults around them.[11]

Too many boys describe receiving sexts from girls as "I know I can get it from" and say that sexting is common only for girls with slut reputations. At the same time, boys also say that girls who don't sext are "stuck up" or "prudish." Boys themselves, on the other hand, are generally not judged on whether or not they sext, and they are often considered heroes if they acquire and distribute sexts, particularly those considered hard to get. Hello, it's 1959 calling—they want their old-fashioned double standard back.

Outside of the legal concerns, that's where the troubling issues about sexting lie: the terrible pressure American girls feel to create and distribute erotic selfies, using their sexuality to prove their worth or enhance their popularity. The performance of eroticism, Peggy Orenstein calls it in her new book *Girls & Sex: Navigating the Complicated New Landscape* (2016),[12] too often disconnected from girls' sense of who they are, what they want, and who they want to be. And Orenstein sees this as a common prelude to the modern young woman's performance of sex itself—something done for an audience (males), not for the woman's own pleasure or self-expression.

The best response isn't to forbid sexting—it's for adults to talk with girls and boys about sexuality and pleasure, mutuality and responsibility.

THE MEDIA AND THE LAW: SYMBIOTIC PANIC PROMOTERS

The media's exploitative response to sexting has focused on titillation and agony, driving America's anxiety about it. The media love stories about sexting, because it gives them a chance to talk about sex, to show young women on screen looking attractive, and to invite viewers/readers to speculate about all the sex teens are having.

If you doubt this, watch any TV news story on sexting with the sound *off.* Teasers before the story and intercuts during the story are invariably salacious. The same dynamic holds with "news" stories of prostitutes (arrested or murdered, it makes no difference), stories of students having sex with teachers, zoning conflicts regarding strip clubs, and allegations of sexual violence. It's all a media opportunity to showcase sex, with the self-righteous, ain't-it-awful deniability of "It's news, and people have a right to know."

Whether the story involves pleasure or exploitation, the media love a sex story. And the media write the sexting story to include both.

And so periodically we hear of a case in which a couple of kids are arrested—scholarships lost, futures ruined—invariably described as the kids' fault. Occasionally we hear about sexting "rings," which "infect" schools and throw communities into a panic—as in Cañon City, Colorado, for example, recently involving some 100 students from a single high school. Parents report being shocked; law enforcement says it is overwhelmed by the task of sorting through mountains of digital "evidence."[13] That alone should tell us how normative sexting is, and how unnecessarily hysterical common adult reactions are.

America's legal response to sexting has been the equivalent of using nuclear weapons to punish littering. In 30 states, sexting is legally described as the creation and distribution of child pornography, among the most serious felonies there are. Bizarrely, these laws say the same young person can be both a victim and a perpetrator. It defines a moonstruck (or bragging) boyfriend as a snarling predator. So laws that were designed to protect children's lives are now being used to destroy them. It's the worst possible case of burning down the house to roast a pig.

Depending on the state and on circumstances, kids (boys or girls) who have taken or sent a nude selfie and kids (boys or girls) who have them on their phones can be prosecuted as felons, jailed, and possibly forced to register for life as sex offenders. Especially at the local level, this issue is tailor-made for salacious law enforcement officials who burn with fear and ignorance of sexual behavior. Egged on by a cultural obsession with child pornography and highly exaggerated stranger danger, law enforcement has generally responded with the bluntest instruments it has.

As Louisa County (VA) prosecutor Rusty McGuire said about nude selfies possibly going beyond where they were intended, "What do you do? Turn a blind eye? You're letting teenagers incite the prurient interest of predators around the country," fueling a demand that "can only be met by the actual abuse of real children."[14]

What total nonsense. As a professional, McGuire should know better, but apparently doesn't: "The conjecture that the Internet or sexting has increased the number of molesters or their motivation to offend has not really been supported by the evidence," says David Finkelhor. He adds that U.S. rates of child molesting and sexual offenses in general have declined since sexting has become popular.[15]

When kids are busted for sexting, they often respond, "Yeah, I know I shouldn't do it. . . ." But they never say, "Yeah, I knew I could go to jail for a thousand years, but I decided to do it anyway." Studies invariably show that a majority of teens are flabbergasted at this latter possibility.[16] It's similar to their response to age-of-consent laws. When kids are busted for having under-age sex, they say they know they're not supposed to do it, but never say they knew they were risking arrest and imprisonment.

You can understand that when teens' lived experience is that they can drive, have a job, get contraception, control their own spending money, and have intense sexual feelings, they assume they own their bodies. But our society's consensus is that young people don't control, and can't delegate control, of their sexuality (that prerogative belongs primarily to America's retail sector, which shamelessly exploits teens' bodies as part of advertising). If our society is going to selectively commandeer teens' bodies until they're 18, we need to explain that bizarre fact to them much more effectively: legally, there can be no visual record of the sexuality of minors.

As Marsha Levick, co-founder of the nonprofit Juvenile Law Center, says of sexting, "Grownups fear that their kids are doing things they don't understand. [But] kids are finding a normal part of adolescent experimentation being criminalized."[17]

Real child pornography is a record of child abuse. Sexting is generally a record of adolescent hijinks, which sometimes go awry. Lumping the two together reflects adult anxiety about young people's sexuality, not a sophisticated understanding of it. Arresting these kids for the creation, possession, or distribution of child pornography is a perversion of the law. It turns the 15-year-old who poses into both a victim and a perpetrator. How exactly is justice served by arresting these kids?

By watering down the definition of "child pornography," such laws undermine our attempts to reduce the actual sexual exploitation of children, and to catch and treat those who would really harm our kids.

Ironically, the campaign against sexting holds kids to a higher standard of judgment than adults. With adults, we generally don't criminalize poor judgment unless it involves coercion or demonstrable harm. If you take nude photos of your wife and then share them with a friend the day after your divorce, she can call you a bastard (which you would be), but she can't sue you. She certainly can't get you on a sex offender registry that lumps you in with rapists and child molesters.

Fortunately, laws regulating sexting have already been changed in over a dozen states, often dramatically reducing the negative consequences of teen sexting and giving prosecutors some discretion. But even these states still fail to distinguish between consensual sexting and deliberate attempts to harm and humiliate. They still criminalize private, consensual sexting between teens, which is unfortunate—and focuses blame on the sexting rather than violations of consent.

Those who say we need draconian laws to discourage kids from sexting need a reality check—they simply don't work. Both science and everyday experience tell us that the Abstinence Model ("just say no, because we say so") does not work with teens. Demanding that they stop sexting hasn't prevented them from sexting, and it won't. Do you remember the laws of the '60s and '70s that made felons of pot smokers? They didn't reduce pot smoking, they just destroyed tens of thousands of lives. Many of those people still languish in jail.[18]

So what should parents do?

Just like you don't want the first sex talk you have with your kids to be about pornography, you also don't want it to be about sexting. So put this book down and go talk with each of your kids about sexuality. Any aspect of it. Make the subject the newest part of the family's ongoing vocabulary. You can return to the topic of sexting soon after.

So what do you say to kids about sexting?

Start by asking questions. What are kids around school doing with their devices? Have them show you their phone and their latest apps. Are they using Kik Messenger (texting for free, with no record)? Instagram (enables public photos and private chat)? Tumblr? Vine (homemade six-second video clips—maybe of you)? Because they live on their phones, you want their mobile activity acknowledged and discussed as part of the family's life.

And then the complex part begins: the larger, long-term conversation about gender, consent, and the power of sexuality in young peoples' lives. Because without this context, your conversation about sexting will soon come down to "don't do it, it's dangerous." And they'll say OK, and that will be the end of the conversation. Net influence on your kid: close to zero. The Abstinence Model doesn't work with sex, and it won't work with sexting.

The common advice parents get about sexting is to persuade kids about its dangers: how it supposedly invites predators into their lives, how it can ruin their reputation, how college reps or potential employers will see the images, how you can't control what happens to the pictures once you hit "send"—because the Internet, unlike love, is forever.[19]

The predator part is extremely rare, and the rest of it contains some truth—but that's only part of the story. And to an adolescent, it isn't the most interesting part of the story. Because for teens, sexting is part of an intricate dance of courtship, peer pressure, popularity measurement, and expressions of passion, autonomy, body ownership, intimacy, competitiveness, and impulsivity.

What do you tell your son who wants to collect as many nude selfies as his buddies? What do you tell your daughter who wants to prove she loves her boyfriend? What do you tell your teen who calls a classmate a slut or a player? "Just say no" doesn't work—and doesn't prepare them for the complicated situations they're in or soon will be.

And what about the ethics of consent—why *not* pass along a nude selfie of someone when it will get you prestige with your pals? And besides, didn't she ask for it by taking and sending the picture? That's when you talk about consent, about ownership, and about violating someone's privacy or trust. Teens are capable of moral reasoning at a higher level than "Don't do it because I'll kill you" or "Don't do it because you could get in a lot of trouble." Talking about how you want your teen to see other human beings is what this is mostly about. Talking about how sexuality is the coin of the realm in adolescence is the rest of what it's about. If you don't talk about these, you can't talk about sexting effectively.

So here are some topics that form the context for teen sexting. Yes, any reasonable parent would have trouble discussing these with their teen—and yet if you want to influence your kids' sexting behavior, this is what you need to talk about:

• The excitement of being desired
• The excitement of being attractive, and fear that you're not
• How to express yourself erotically without genital involvement; how to express yourself sexually without intercourse
• Sexual pleasure
• The fact that masturbation is OK
• What to do if you're in love and you feel pressured
• What to do if you're in love and can't decide what to do
• What to do if you're dying to see what girls look like nude
• What to do if you're looking at adult porn and feeling troubled
• Why being respectful to others is a good way to live
• "Let's face it, some boys (or girls) think you're hot"
• Under what circumstances would someone like you sext?

Most parents don't like to have their kids' sexuality pushed in their face. And yet in the 21st century, that's pretty much where it is. *That's our problem as parents, not theirs as kids.*

Discovering a nude selfie on your kid's phone can be extremely upsetting. Online safety websites contradict each other with their advice on this, from "destroy the pictures" to "save the pictures," from "contact the school" to "contact the authorities" to "contact other parents."

If you're suddenly in this situation, the specific circumstances matter greatly. They may involve state or federal laws, possible "Romeo and Juliet" exemptions, various levels of mandatory reporting requirements, and possible formal investigations.[20] Naively trying to do the right thing can still get you or your child in a lot of trouble; there's serious tension between deleting potential evidence in a criminal case and preserving evidence that can be, itself, illegal. Even contacting another parent may have unintended consequences for you or your child.

Given the culturally radioactive response to teen nudity and sexuality, any institution you deal with (school, law enforcement, child protective services, etc.) regarding actual sexting will care much more about protecting its own bureaucratic butt than anything else (such as your family's welfare). Thus, the only reasonable thing to do if you find nude selfies on your child's phone is to contact an experienced lawyer immediately, and to take the phone out of circulation.

By all means, tell your child that if he or she receives a nude selfie, regardless of who it's from,

1. S/he should tell you immediately; and
2. S/he must not forward it to anyone else. *Really.*

And then you and your child need to have a series of talks about the issue—what s/he thinks has happened, how s/he feels, what s/he needs now.

America's problem isn't sexting—it's how we raise kids, marginalize sexuality, teach boys to disrespect girls, teach girls to use sex to attract boys, and then hesitate to talk with them about the results. We then have very few tools left—and they're basically all nuclear weapons. And so in America, we destroy teens' lives in order to save them.

Chapter Six

COUPLES' CONFLICTS ABOUT PORN—INNOVATIVE APPROACHES

Marco looks at porn. His wife Lila knows this and hates it. In fact, she has withdrawn from him sexually because of her resentment—or, as she puts it, because of "his porn-whores."

Travis looks at porn. His wife Mona accuses him of infidelity. She says he needs to "choose" between her and "your other girlfriends."

James looks at porn. His girlfriend Petra says she knows he thinks about beautiful young porn actresses while they have sex, and that now she feels self-conscious about undressing in front of him or having sex with the lights on.

Sam looks at porn. He wants his wife Yuko to do oral, to let him ejaculate in her mouth, and then dribble it down her chin. She's willing to do oral, but he thrusts too deeply. She's not wild about him ejaculating in her mouth. She certainly doesn't want jiz on her chin, or anywhere else. So they don't do oral.

Aaron looks at porn. He and his wife Esther have sex only three or four times a year. He watches porn. She doesn't. She's resentful that he has an almost-daily sex life and she doesn't.

Jason looks at porn. He's lost interest in LaKayla sexually. He looks forward to masturbating with porn in the mornings, when she leaves for work before he does.

As a therapist, it's difficult to sit through these porn-related cases week after week. The level of shame, guilt, anger, and suffering people go through is heartbreaking. I believe a lot of the suffering is completely unnecessary, which in some ways makes this work even harder.

This is a difficult chapter to write for the same reason: the level of pain and unnecessary suffering I need to address.

* * *

There are two fundamental arguments couples have about porn:

1. "Watching porn is not OK." *"Yes it is."*
2. "Watching porn leads to consequences that are not OK: a) for you; b) for me; c) for our couple; d) for our kids." *"Maybe when other guys watch, but not me."*

Across America, the conversation has shifted substantially from argument #1 to argument #2. And so when couples are in conflict about porn, the non-consumer who 40 years ago used to say, "I don't want you watching porn because I think it's garbage, it's wrong, and it's bad," now more typically says, "I don't want you watching porn because it has results I don't want—and you shouldn't, either."

* * *

When I train therapists to deal with this subject, I say, "How would you handle the cases involving porn if you dealt with them the same way you deal with every other couples conflict? Or to put it a different way, if you handle couples differently when the subject is porn, why?"

Many therapists find these questions disturbing. And if therapists are treating conflicts about porn differently than they treat other cases, it should. Because it's treating porn conflicts differently than other marital conflicts that sucks a couple into trouble in the first place. If therapists duplicate that mistake in their treatment there's a limit to how helpful they can be.

* * *

When couples argue about whether someone did or didn't do something wrong by watching porn, I have to ask about the couple's contract. Did the porn consumer break an agreement he made to not watch porn? Does the non-consumer have the right to invoke an agreement that she thinks should exist, but the couple didn't create? Does the non-consumer have the right to demand an agreement covering future behavior?

When people say "let's live together" or "let's get married," they generally don't discuss enough of the details. Maybe they know they'll have a dog, or that they definitely won't have a dog. Maybe they've discussed whether and how many kids they'll have (although a shocking number of couples don't, and then spend years in heartbreaking conflict about it).

Couples usually (though not always) tell each other that they expect monogamy—but they rarely discuss what this includes. Ex-boyfriend via

Facebook? Masturbating with a stranger in a chatroom? Skype sex with someone you pay? Sending (or receiving) a topless photo? A massage with a happy ending?

Pornography is part of that vague undiscussed arena. OK to watch? OK to watch and masturbate? OK to pay someone who strips or masturbates on a webcam? OK to watch and masturbate an hour before or after we have sex? Do romance novels count as porn? What about "erotica" like *Fifty Shades of Grey*?

* * *

Many women are troubled about their mate watching porn. They variously insist it means:

- He doesn't love me
- He doesn't care about my feelings
- He wishes he were with someone else
- He's going to have an affair, or is having an affair (or watching porn *is* an affair)

Of course, it's fairly easy to check on these very upsetting assumptions. Unfortunately, many women don't. Some don't bother because they won't believe the answers they get. Understandably, their mates feel angry that they're being told how they feel without their input. This contributes to the distance both partners soon feel. And the assumptions remain in place, hurting both of them.

With a consistently negative narrative, the PornPanic encourages women to believe things about their partner's porn use like:

- It's about me personally
- It causes our problems, and is therefore (1) my business, and (2) irresponsible behavior
- I know what my partner thinks/feels about porn, and I know how it affects him
- I know I'm not desirable enough to compete with porn images

These interpretations make his porn-watching her business. She decides she has the moral high ground from which to dictate what his problem is, the fact that he must get it fixed, and what the treatment needs to be.

In addition, her narrative, supported by today's anti-porn, Public Danger culture, is:

- Interest in porn is not normal
- Use of porn is selfish
- I have a right to ban it from our life and my home

Like pouring gasoline on a destructive fire, today's PornPanic delegitimizes men's interest in porn, and legitimizes women's pain about their partner's porn use, no matter how unreasonable her feelings are. That's how moral panics work—like the satanic abuse scare of the 1980s, in which adults believed things that couldn't possibly have happened, sending innocent people to jail and destroying the lives of thousands of children. The therapy profession, unfortunately, is mostly under the same PornPanic spell as the general public.

SOLVING THE PROBLEM TOO SOON?
SOLVING THE WRONG PROBLEM?

"I want you to stop watching porn" is a solution to a problem.

The question is, what is the problem that this solution is designed to address?

Some people do think that porn, or watching porn, is disgusting or wrong. If so, "less porn" definitely sounds like the solution. In couples, this can set up a confrontation of needs: B wants A watching less porn (frequently *no* porn), while A likes to watch porn (and doesn't like being told what to do). What will they do? Couples rarely approach this situation as a collaborative team, so things usually degenerate into emotional pushing and shoving. I often see these power struggles in my office—either when he refuses to stop watching, or when he agrees to stop watching, and then gets caught watching. Again.

(Memo to besieged men—do not promise to stop watching porn unless you're 100 percent certain that you will. Not 99 percent; *100 percent.* Can't be that sure? Then don't promise. If necessary, quarrel instead—in the long run, that's better.)

So if she wants distance from porn and he wants it in his life, how are they going to reconcile this? I now deal with this situation every week. It's interesting just how much of a sense of entitlement these aggrieved wives and girlfriends have—as if porn is somehow different than anything else they'd quarrel over as equals.

I don't tell couples that porn is good, and I don't even say watching it is OK. But I do ask what kind of relationship they want—one in which people make demands and tell each other how it's going to be, or a more collaborative arrangement in which two people work together to resolve their difficulties.

That said, "I want you to stop watching porn" can be an imagined solution to specific (though unspoken) grievances:

- I'm upset that we don't have sex anymore (or hardly ever)
- I don't feel desired
- I don't like my body

- I'm afraid you don't like my body
- I'm afraid you're having an affair or might have an affair
- I'm uncomfortable with our kids' budding sexuality
- I feel out of control of my life or our marriage
- I don't want you having sexual pleasure without me
- I'm afraid you might start looking at our kids' friends in a creepy way

If someone is struggling with any of these feelings, she (or he) deserves to be heard and comforted and should have their feelings addressed.

However, someone demanding that her (or his) mate stop watching porn may or may not even be aware of these feelings, as they can be very uncomfortable. A good marital citizen is committed to understanding his or her feelings so they can advocate for what they actually need, rather than settle for quarrelling that can't get them what they need.

So when someone says they want their partner to stop watching porn, I ask if they have a specific complaint about how their partner treats them (for example, calling them the wrong name during sex, or continually teasing them about the size of their breasts). If they do, I suggest we discuss the complaint without assuming we know the cause; while it might be related to porn, it might not be.

Whether a behavior under discussion is about sex or not, starting the discussion by arguing over a solution is a mistake—negotiating solutions is the *last* step a couple should take, not the first. If your complaint is phrased as, "I hate the way you're always telling me my butt is too big, so I want you to stop watching porn," you and your mate will predictably argue about porn, and the issue of you feeling disrespected and pushed away will get lost—along with any sympathy he may have about you feeling hurt.

So how does this work in real life?

She complains he's a porn addict. He says he's not. She says anyone who watches that much must be addicted. He says he's not. She says, "I want you to get treatment for your porn addiction"; she may threaten consequences such as humiliation or even divorce if he refuses. He doesn't want to get treated for something he doesn't consider a problem. She says, "If you won't address my anguish it just proves that porn is more important to you than I am; in fact, since you say you love me but won't stop, you must be addicted."

He feels cornered, and like anyone who feels cornered about anything, he fights back, maybe gets nasty, and certainly isn't cooperative. And he definitely doesn't address the pain she must be in if she's making statements and demands like these.

When this couple comes into therapy they often want me to adjudicate whether or not he watches "too much" porn or is even a porn addict. They're typically surprised and disappointed when I won't do that. I've learned that doing so is pointless, because no matter what I say, one of them will almost certainly reject my verdict.

"Let's put that question aside for a moment," I often respond instead, "and pursue some other questions that might be more helpful." I could ask, "What do you mean by porn addiction?" I could also ask, "Well, if you're not addicted, why do you keep doing something you know upsets her?" But those questions aren't helpful, either. In fact, they can obscure the real issue.

Instead, I'd rather ask her, "Other than watching porn, what is he doing or not doing sexually, or in your relationship, that you dislike?"

In response to that question, women often say things like

- He won't look at me during sex
- He calls me the wrong name during sex
- He wants me to dress too sexy in bed, around the house, or out in public
- He teases me or criticizes my body in mean ways
- He won't initiate sex
- He won't have sex with me at all
- He's constantly asking for sex
- He loses his erection or comes too quickly with me
- He can't ejaculate when we have sex (or can't ejaculate inside me)
- He asks for totally outlandish things (e.g., anal, threesomes, watch me with another girl) that he should know I won't do
- He looks at women on the street in creepy ways
- He looks at our teen daughter's friends in creepy ways

Many people would feel bad about having to deal with any of these things. In fact, I deal with these and similar complaints in couples therapy all the time. When I begin treatment, I never assume I know what the cause is, whether it's porn, a broken heart, major depression, someone having been molested, an endocrine problem, a deep lack of empathy, or something else.

"So let's pursue these problems as far as we can without assuming we know what the cause is, and see where we end up," I say. "If it turns out that porn is driving behaviors you don't like, we can definitely address that." Sometimes it is, often it isn't.

This approach deemphasizes the porn aspect of a situation and emphasizes the actual lived experience of the people involved—particularly their pain. Rather than starting with a solution (no more porn) based on a hypothesis (porn causes your behavior which gives me pain) that may not be accurate, I'd rather start in the other direction: Your behavior gives me pain, and I'd like to figure out what we can do about this. Maybe I'll find out what drives your behavior, and maybe I won't; if you can change it in a genuine way without me fully understanding how you did so, I can live with that.

The trick here is to get the couple actually cooperating in her articulating her pain (as well as his, of course)—not to hurt him or to prove a point, but to share information with a partner. And the trick here is to get him to listen—not because he's misbehaved and has to take his medicine, not because her diagnosis of him is right and he has to be bludgeoned into accepting it, but because his partner is sharing information that he needs and should want.

It may take weeks or months of therapy to maneuver the two of them into that collaborative space together. When they are, the question of whether he's a porn addict often goes away, as does a lot of his defensiveness; what's left is, "Omigosh, we have an issue here, you're upset, what are we gonna do? Please tell me more." "OK, I'll tell you more." My job is to keep the sharing cooperative and productive, rather than hostile, blaming, judging, defensive, repetitive, or superficial.

Does he want her to feel belittled, pushed away, unattractive? Generally not. Now the next trick: Don't let them look for a solution too quickly, which often ends up with him saying, "I'm certainly not giving up x." Instead, I want him curious and caring. I want him expressing sympathy—preferably on his own, or with help from me if he needs it. I also want her perceiving that he cares about her, completely independent of whatever his porn consumption is.

There's something quite lovely about this process—a hurt person behaves like a partner, a defensive person behaves like a partner, and their curiosity has a healing effect. Once that healing balm starts soothing them both, spontaneous apologies often come. Eventually we can have the next conversation—Honey, I hate to see you so upset, what can we do about this (whatever "this" is)? Or: Honey, I can see a little private time works for you, how can we make that happen?

* * *

As couples therapy unfolds and people can create a collaborative mood on their own, we're ready to address specific complaints: you keep asking for anal sex even though I keep saying I'll never do that; you don't seem to like my body anymore; and so on. These are hard subjects for people to discuss, but it's necessary. If you have that kind of complaint, addressing it honestly gives you a better chance of success rather than trying to get your partner to stop looking at porn. Similarly, if you've stopped having sex because it's boring and you watch a lot of porn and your partner wants you to stop, talking about sex instead of talking about porn gives you a better chance to create change.

And that's where the serious difficulty comes in: talking about sex honestly. I'm very sympathetic about this, because it can be so painful. But without honest talk about sex, it's rare that the sexual relationship will change. You can talk about porn for a thousand years—but that's not the same as talking about "I don't enjoy sex with you," or "I'm still really hurt about what you said about my body five years ago," or "You don't seem to be thinking about me when we make love," or "I don't like the way you kiss" or "Your inhibitions about your body make it very difficult for me to enjoy sex with you."

If you imagine what it would probably be like to say one of these things to your partner—especially if you love him or her—you can see why people would rather fight about porn than talk honestly about sex. Unfortunately, today's PornPanic gives people the perfect excuse for not talking about sex—by encouraging women to make demands about porn, and encouraging porn consumers to feel guilty, broken, or defiant.

IS PORNOGRAPHY USE A FORM OF INFIDELITY?

This is another common question that I generally don't answer. "Infidelity" is a contract violation. Most couples have extremely short "contracts"—they agree to share money, live together, be nice to each other, and, usually, to be monogamous. People rarely define monogamy while they're coupling up, and when they do they almost never mention pornography.

People can disagree until the end of time about whether looking at pornography is a form of infidelity. When she says, "I don't want you looking at porn because it's a form of infidelity," he usually says, "No it isn't," and then they disagree about that. Her pain doesn't get addressed, because it doesn't get spoken. He doesn't get a chance to be sympathetic, nor does he get a chance to be heard about his interest in masturbation or sexual fantasy.

So when someone says, "You shouldn't look at porn because it's a form of infidelity," I ask what else is the problem with his porn-watching. Sooner or later she will say one of two things:

A. It's wrong, disgusting, or dangerous, and therefore he shouldn't do it, *or*
B. It's involved with other things that I don't like, such as masturbation, violence, casual sex, oral sex, or women with perfect bodies.

Either way, we can then discuss the couple's problem without having to decide about "infidelity." If it really is (A), it raises an interesting question: What do you two do when you disagree on what's immoral or wrong? If it's (B), we go back to the process I described previously, in which we focus on the lived experience of feeling hurt, rejected, left out, or unimportant (or sympathetic, dismayed, or embarrassed), without assuming we know the root cause and therefore the solution.

Anyone can decide that virtually anything is a form of infidelity; after all, the definition of infidelity is completely subjective. Does it include flirting with strangers at the airport? Kissing a co-worker at a party? Getting a lap dance while on a business trip to Boston? You won't have any trouble finding someone with either opinion about each of these.

Some people say that looking at porn constitutes infidelity because it means someone is experiencing their eroticism outside of the couple. That's a definition that challenges adult autonomy in a serious way. It also raises the question: Is masturbation a form of infidelity? Because masturbating—with or without porn, with or without fantasy—is indeed experiencing one's eroticism outside of the couple. If that's unacceptable, then porn is the least of it—it's masturbating that's the problem.

For anyone who says, "Well, fantasy is in the imagination, but porn involves real people," I'd say two things:

1. The porn consumer's relationship is not with a person, it's with a character played by an actress; and
2. People can have that same fantasy relationship with Jennifer Lopez, a college-age neighbor, or Florence Nightingale, whether or not one looks at a media image of them.

The consumption of porn doesn't involve relating to the person of the actress—her worries about health insurance, her delight that her kid got accepted to Vanderbilt, her hope of getting a part on Broadway—any more than our consumption of an NFL game involves relating to the person of Tom Brady—his marital concerns, his kids' health, or his feelings about getting older. We care about the character Brady plays—an NFL quarterback—and to the extent that he does that poorly, we abandon him immediately.

By the way, loving gossip about a celebrity does *not* constitute caring about them. Pick a political figure you *hate*—say, Hillary Clinton or Donald Trump. Your interest in gossip about that person is an interest in the commodity (including popular conflict about) called Hillary or The Donald. Wanting to feel connected to the current story about these consumer products doesn't mean we care about the people—or, for that matter, our country's future.

IF SOMEONE CLAIMS THE BIBLE SAYS USING PORN IS INFIDELITY

There are several key passages from the New Testament and Proverbs that appear to condemn pornography[1]—if that's how someone wants to interpret them. Of course, if someone wants Biblical justification for opposing virtually any sexual expression, it's easy to find. You could even read the erotic Song of Songs as a satire "(Kiss me with the kisses of your mouth . . ."—oh puh-leeze!), or decide that the passage praising Lot's daughters for seducing him was written by Satan.

The Bible was written in a time of radical gender separation and powerful traditions of proper gender-based behavior. Children were a valued economic resource, and so many women died (or become infertile) during childbirth that multiple wives were common. In most ancient societies women had few rights, and most Middle Eastern cultures were obsessed with menstrual impurity (many still are).

So the meaning of infidelity, flirting, perversion, and masturbation were very, very different then than they are now. And of course there are some barbaric practices in the Bible, including capital punishment for adultery. So everyone who wants the Bible in their lives has to make peace with it in their own way. But nobody—nobody—believes every single thing in the Bible literally, whether it's an elderly woman giving birth, or the suggestion of selling one's daughter into slavery, or the way that menstruating women make furniture unclean. If, during conflict with one's mate, people of faith would admit that they want what they want, rather than using Scripture to justify what they want, those couples would have more productive conflict.

POWER STRUGGLES

Perhaps because they're a familiar part of our lives from childhood on, many people underestimate the damage that power struggles bring to a relationship. When one person says, "If you love me, you'll do x," it doesn't matter what x is—making a person prove they love you, and dictating the terms thereof, is just bad for relationships. It engenders bad feelings in the person who acquiesces, or in the person who doesn't get what they want. It becomes part of the couple's history, and it will be used again.

When people in a couple tell each other what they have to do or are forbidden to do, the subject is no longer the thing being discussed—it's power. When one person says I know you better than you know yourself, the subject is power. When one person says, "Here's the condition under which I'll stay"—or be loving, or have sex—the subject is power. When one person says, "I get to make the definitions around here" of terms like infidelity, addiction, masculinity, sex, and intimacy, the subject is power.

And when one person says, "I have a feeling about you, and although it's contradicted by what you say or by actual evidence, I'm going to continue to believe my feeling"—the subject is power.

People don't like hearing this. People accuse me of taking sides. And I do take sides, although not in the way they think. I'm on the side of collaborative decision-making, rather than one person dictating terms to the other. I'm on the side of adults having dignity and autonomy. I'm on the side of adults treating each other respectfully.

Perhaps it's easier to see this when the subject is something other than pornography. For example, imagine a husband telling his wife, "I've had it with your knitting—you're out every Tuesday at the knitting club! You get two, three knitting magazines in the mail every month! Your closets are filled with wool of every imaginable color! There's even knitting needles in the kitchen! I absolutely forbid you from knitting anymore!"

The wife may be a little over the top about knitting, and the husband's anger is understandable—but would you think this is a reasonable response? What about someone who tells their boyfriend or girlfriend, "I forbid you from watching TV shows featuring racial stereotypes. They're bad for society, and there's no place for them in our home." Or, "You may not eat veal, whether you're with me or not. They treat those little calves horribly in order to produce tender veal, and I will not have either one of us supporting such a cruel industry."

Whether we sympathize with one mate or the other in these vignettes, it should be clear that one person making unilateral demands or decisions undermines the relationship—often creating more problems than it solves. That kind of power grab is no more helpful—or intimate, or respectful—when the topic is pornography.

When couples quarrel, they frequently invoke common ideas from popular culture, including references to what's normal. Asserting that you know what's normal and that you judge that your partner isn't—the subject of that conversation is power.

For example, sometimes we live in a time or place when slow dancing with someone else's husband is considered scandalous; in other cultural circumstances it's acceptable. This is completely different from the question of how you feel when you see or hear that your wife is slow dancing with another man. If you feel bad about it you deserve sympathy and a caring conversation with your wife. But if the conversation is about whether or not your feelings are normal, you're unlikely to feel satisfied, and each of you is unlikely to feel understood.

We live in a time in which porn addiction is a popular idea. Popular culture also has plenty of ideas about normal amounts of sex in marriage, normal amounts of masturbation, normal sexual fantasies, and whether someone's pain about being forbidden to masturbate is equivalent to their partner's pain about them masturbating. When it comes to sex in general and porn in particular, too many psychologists simply adopt our culture's ideas of what's normal, and proclaim that to be truth or human nature. Both Dr. Phil and Oprah Winfrey got rich, powerful, and famous telling people—mostly women—what's normal, and encouraging them to demand that their loved ones behave in so-called normal ways.

The real answer to a power struggle is to acknowledge it and to agree to address substantive issues rather than attempt to win, be right, or get the other person to submit. Yes, this requires self-discipline, communication, patience, tolerance, and a real desire to create a working partnership. Struggling for power is much easier. Of course, people who struggle for power in relationships are generally not happy with the result—whether they win *or* lose.

So you can say you don't like porn without having to demonize porn-watching as abnormal. On the other hand, calling porn-watching abnormal or saying your boyfriend's favorite porn is perverse isn't a good enough reason for him to stop watching it. After all, he may not agree that his activities are abnormal or perverse. The two of you could disagree about that until the end of time.

You're much better off talking about feeling left out or insecure about your body (or whatever is troubling you about his porn-watching) than you are talking about what's wrong with his porn-watching. The first will draw him to you, while the second will create an adversarial situation.

This is the perfect place to say clearly that not every problem involving porn is a porn problem—just like not every problem involving a car is a car problem. For example, if your husband borrows your car and it gets dented while he's parked downtown, then he tries to hide it from you or deny that it happened while he had the car, that's *not* a car problem, right? That's a problem of selfishness, dishonesty, fear, or something else.

And so similarly, it's not a "porn problem" if:

- He leaves porn accessible to the kids
- He leaves evidence of his masturbation around the house
- He talks about porn way more than you want to hear
- He makes lots of jokes about porn or sex that you don't find funny
- He spends more money on porn than your household budget can support
- He says he doesn't care that you're unhappy about his porn use
- He periodically demands that you watch porn with him after you've said you don't want to
- He says he's not interested in how you feel about his porn-watching

Therefore, attempting to address these aggravating or hurtful situations by demanding he stop watching porn will be of little value. This is another way that both today's PornPanic and the Porn Addiction movement actually undermine relationships: by assuming that all behavior involving pornography is primarily about pornography, and by assuming that people who behave poorly are under the influence of pornography, rather than the more powerful explanation that they're making choices that correspond to their needs and values, their internal strengths and weaknesses.

COMPETING WITH PORN STARS

Porn or no porn, every man and woman has to figure out how to feel OK with themselves when they don't look as good as others, have as much money as others, or have children as well-behaved as others. This is the fundamental existential task of all people who want to enjoy life, and porn didn't invent it.

How do you get through the day, comparing your income to Mark Zuckerberg's, your home to Martha Stewart's, your influence to Oprah Winfrey's, your golf game to Lydia Ko's, and your body to, well, any 25-year-old movie star's? This isn't a female problem or a male problem, it's a human problem.

If your partner watches porn, that's just one more opportunity to either compare yourself unfavorably, or to work on that darn inescapable, internal existential project.

Do keep in mind that men who watch porn are not relating to the actresses—they're relating to the characters the actresses play. Porn consumers don't care any more about the people who make porn than sports fans care about the athletes who play sports. We cheer, we groan, we wager, we play in fantasy leagues (you understand we're talking about sports, not porn, right?), we swear off a certain player or team.

And at the end of the day, which of us cares about LeBron James or Missy Franklin or Tiger Woods? We consume them the same way we consume porn stars. In particular, we consume their bodies and performances. When they can't provide these to our satisfaction anymore, we discard them. The same is true of musicians, stage actors, and all other performers. We don't care how cellists might be sacrificing their wrists, or stage actors their families. As long as Yo-Yo Ma and Hilary Swank can perform for us, we consume them. When they can't, we drop them. Paradoxically, the most beloved performers are the least human to us.

I'm not saying this is good (or bad). It's just that porn actresses aren't the only people we objectify, valuing them only for their performance and body, rather than for their humanity. If watching porn encourages objectification of performers and performances we value, so does watching sports. And the next time you treat the supermarket checker as an extension of the scanning machine rather than as a person whose kid might be sick or whose husband might be unemployed, ask yourself how different that is from watching a porn star (who just may be making more money than the supermarket checker).

Now some people *do* mind their partner watching Tom Brady or LeBron James too enthusiastically. He gets jealous when she says, "Wow, look at LeBron's muscles," or "Wow, that Tom Brady sure has guts." She gets jealous when he says, "That Serena has cleavage to die for." Yes, some people feel threatened when their partner appreciates a public figure's body—which is another way of saying, "I compare myself and don't like what I see." Don't blame your partner when you put yourself in that position.

The ultimate issue in many couples in conflict about pornography is the decline or disappearance of their once-enjoyable sex life. This is extremely hard for couples to discuss, given the shame, grief, confusion, rejection, failure, and hopelessness that people often feel.

As a therapist, I can tell you that sitting through that conversation, and even encouraging people to reveal more of their heartache, is very, very painful. It's particularly poignant because there's no guarantee that acknowledging the depth of the problem and the depth of the pain will lead to a satisfying solution. What we do know is that without conversations like that, meaningful change will almost certainly not occur. And emotional separation, perhaps with quiet resentment, will continue. While it's common to say that porn consumers are selfish and rejecting of their partners, a lot of porn use is actually a desperate attempt to stay in a sexually unfulfilling couple.

If couples could talk about sex honestly and directly, most antagonistic conversations about pornography would just go away. Some couples would have more sex. Others wouldn't, but conflict about porn would no longer be all that interesting.

SO AM I TAKING HIS SIDE?

When I approach couples' conflicts about porn in this way, people sometimes ask this question. That in itself is interesting—that a balanced approach, an approach that sees each partner's pain as equally valid, that sees the couple as the unit that needs healing rather than seeing one individual who needs to be fixed (while the other needs healing), can be seen as biased.

As a rule, marriage counselors are trained to see couples in pain, rather than seeing one victim and one victimizer (the exception is domestic violence). And yet when I propose to use that very same proven approach when there's conflict about porn, I am sometimes accused of "taking his side." Similarly, when I don't see the porn as the problem, but rather see that there's a couple who doesn't have an existing agreement about something, has an unsatisfying sex life, and is blaming each other for their distress, I'm often accused of "taking his side"—as if he and the porn are co-conspirators, and she's left out.

If I were to say that it were all her fault—the power-tripping, the demands, the inflexibility, the refusal to look at things from his point of view—I'd be accused of taking his side, and that would be accurate. But the same people who would criticize me blaming her for everything somehow expect that I will blame it all on him.

So am I taking his side? No. I'm taking the side of the relationship—a grownup relationship, where each person's interests are valid and must be considered. Her pain about his porn—as serious as it is—is *not* more important than his pain about feeling judged, humiliated, distanced, and told what he can and cannot do. At the same time, his desire for a private life free of her criticism is *not* more important than her pain about feeling excluded, or disrespected, or disenfranchised.

In a situation of high conflict, all feelings are *not* equally reasonable, but all strong feelings must be acknowledged, accepted, and sympathized with before any productive analysis or helpful decisions can be made.

The only way most couples are going to get out of the porn-is-our-problem paradigm is as a mutually compassionate team, not by deciding who is to blame. Getting both to sign on to that approach is step one. It's often the biggest step of all.

Case A

RACHEL & JACKSON: PORN AS INFIDELITY (OR, YOU THOUGHT IT = YOU DID IT)

She was 100 percent sure he was being unfaithful, and it was driving her crazy.

And that was driving him crazy, so he came to see me.

What was Rachel so upset about? "I watch porn," said her husband Jackson. And? "She hates it, says it makes her feel distant from me, says it proves I'm insecure and that I don't love her, don't love anyone but myself."

So what did Jackson want from me? "Tell me how to get her to calm down." This is a pretty common request in therapy: Tell me how to change my partner so my life will be better. Or tell me how to get my partner off my back. Or tell me how to convince my partner that I'm OK. (And as a bonus, help me convince my partner they're wrong.)

In that sense, Jackson's request was immediately familiar, even without the details. "Your situation sounds difficult," I said. "But I can't do remote-control therapy. We can spend most of our time talking about you. Or we can do couples therapy. But we can't operate on Rachel from here if she's across town."

He seemed to appreciate that. So we talked about him, at least for the present session. This bright, good-looking, professionally successful man was sad, lonely, embarrassed, and feeling hopeless. What a contrast these two sides of him were. The contrast centered on the ongoing conflict with his wife, whom he loved.

As Jackson unfolded his story, it included a few stops at a local strip club last year (Rachel knew and resented), a few massages with "happy endings" two years ago (Rachel did not know), and fantasies about other women ("Rachel would kill me if she knew"). "Just for the fantasy?" I asked. "Yes, just for the fantasy," he said. "She's very jealous, and has very strict ideas about monogamy."

Some people still hold the ancient belief that "if you thought it, you did it."[1] Even the sexually austere St. Augustine thanked God for not making him responsible for the content of his dreams; Rachel, apparently, was somewhat less understanding than that. And substantially less wise about the nature of human imagination. Attempting to control our partner's fantasies is one of the more damaging things anyone can do to an intimate relationship.

So Jackson periodically looked at porn (and masturbated, of course), and Rachel hated it. She demanded he stop. Like most men, he agreed. And like most men, he kept looking anyway. He soon got "caught" again. I hate that expression, an adult getting "caught" looking at porn—as if he were a disobedient child, discovered by an angry parent.

Promising he wouldn't watch porn again was a serious mistake. Almost everyone making that promise breaks it, and when they do, they lose the moral equivalence so central in a power struggle. It's one thing for her to say I want you to stop, and for him to say I don't want to stop. At that moment, these people can be equal, with equally legitimate desires. But when he says he'll stop and he doesn't, the issue is no longer about porn. Now it's about him breaking a promise. And he's culpable, even if he felt coerced into promising, and no matter how silly he thinks her feelings are.

"But it was a stupid thing for her to ask. I just said yes to stop the arguing," Jackson complained, wanting sympathy. "Don't you think her demand was ridiculous and controlling?"

"Again, Jackson, rather than talk about her request, let's talk about your response," I reminded him. "You promised something you didn't deliver, right? Doesn't that make you untrustworthy? And if you made a promise you didn't even intend to keep, what should we call that?" Although I asked in a friendly way, the questions still required answers. "You and Rachel can quarrel about whether you are going to watch porn. But it's an entirely different argument when you make a promise, break it, and she resents it."

"I suppose that helps her feel like I'm being unfaithful," he said with a frown. It was a good insight.

I continued asking about Jackson's porn-watching.

Was he comfortable with the content of what he watched? He was. Was he comfortable with the fact that he wanted to watch porn regularly, despite his wife's stated opposition? He was. "It's none of her business," he said. "You sound resentful," I observed. "Yes, of course I am," he replied. "I'm an adult and yet I still have to justify a little relaxation. It's ridiculous."

And how was their sexual relationship—did he enjoy it?

"Not so much," he said, looking away. "Sex used to be pretty good, and we did it most weekends, sometimes more. But you know how things change over time. . . ."

I wanted to know more about these changes, but our time was about up. "Jackson," I said, "we need to decide if you want individual counseling or couples counseling." "Both," he laughed. "I think that's a great idea," I said, "And although I do both, I generally don't do both with the same people. So pick one, and I'll give you a referral for the other."

"Rachel will appreciate you," he said without hesitation. "And although I'd like you as my individual counselor, you can help me find someone good just for myself, right?" I recommended an excellent local colleague. I then gave Jackson my availability for several upcoming weeks, and told him to invite Rachel to call me if she'd agree to come in with him. I also encouraged him to share with his wife as much about our session as he wished. The following day Rachel called, and we quickly made an appointment for two weeks hence.

* * *

And so two weeks later I welcomed Rachel into the office with Jackson. I gave her a chance to tell me about herself, asking about her background, friends, and previous career. They had, in fact, discussed Jackson's recent session, so she was pretty much up to speed. I asked her if we could just dive in and resume where he'd left off, and she agreed.

"Jackson mentioned last week that as the kids grew up, you two starting quarrelling more frequently. Is that how you remember it?" "Yes," she sighed. "We seemed to be growing apart. We periodically fought about the kids—I think I was stricter—or money—he was very concerned about our finances, and often questioned my spending."

At about that time, Jackson was getting increasing recognition at his job (his company makes some kind of computer chip—that's about as technical as I get), and was being given more and more responsibility. He said, "With suppliers in India and customers in the U.K., my workday often included Skype meetings at home, before and after my time in the office. Rachel wasn't very sympathetic."

"But this was just when our two children were really active in high school, needing both of us," she added angrily. "How many of their performances or games did you go to? When did you ever talk with them about their futures?" "Doc, you see what I mean? No sympathy from her." "Dr. Klein, do you see what I mean? No awareness," Rachel responded.

"I imagine this dynamic affected everything around the house—even your sex life," I said quietly. They each studied their shoes. Neither replied.

Long ago, they had agreed that Rachel would be a stay-at-home mom, but as the kids got older, she had less to do and began to mourn their inevitable separation from her. She poured herself into homemaking on their behalf, while trying to "create memories" she imagined they'd treasure after leaving for college. Pretty soon she was driving her teenage kids crazy, wanting validation for her sacrifices and careful planning they hadn't requested. Rachel and Jackson couldn't sympathize with each other's difficulties; they really were looking in very different directions.

And that included different directions sexually. It was easy for her to feel left out, to criticize him, and to imagine all his sexual opportunities: sex workers, affairs, business dinners. She started prying, sometimes becoming aggressive and unreasonable. He felt unfairly accused—"Doc, I didn't have the energy to have an affair, I was working 16-hour days"—and thought she was creating a lot of drama about the family's natural evolution. He started withdrawing from her emotionally, which naturally led to him withdrawing sexually. She did the same; although she craved his attention, her growing mistrust led her to push him away. Ironically, they were cooperatively creating emotional separation without realizing it.

Enter porn.

"Of course, I'd been using it for years," said Jackson. "Yes, and look where it's gotten us," sniped Rachel. I jumped in and interrupted before they could escalate further.

"Wait," I said. "Let's talk about this differently, OK?" They agreed, but it was just a temporary ceasefire, not a respectful understanding.

"Rachel, what exactly is the problem with Jackson looking at porn? I'm not asking you to justify your feelings, I just want to understand them."

And boy, did she have feelings. A real man doesn't watch porn. He was bringing "filth" into their house. He masturbated because he was afraid of impotence with an actual woman (her). Him watching porn proved he had no respect for her. Him watching porn had made him lose interest in her. Him watching porn had made her lose interest in him.

"Do you see how his selfish habit has really damaged our marriage?" she asked.

Actually, I didn't see it that way at all. But I could see that she was terribly distraught. Which I validated—"Rachel, you're obviously very upset about Jackson's porn use." She nodded. "Jackson, I know you love Rachel, so you can be sympathetic when she's upset, even when *you're* what she's upset about, right?" He found the question confusing, as do most people when I first ask this. So I explained. "It's critical that people can sympathize with each other's pain without having to agree with them. Otherwise, as soon as our partner disagrees with us we'd be irrevocably isolated from each other. People could never reconcile about a disagreement, and could never feel cared about during or after a disagreement." I could see them thinking this over.

"I guess the technical term for this is 'empathy,'" I said matter-of-factly. "I'll give you a chance to practice this for homework." They agreed.

"A second thing I want to discuss is the important principle of not solving a problem too soon. You both know that from your professional work, right?" They did. "Rachel, 'Jackson not watching porn' is a solution to a problem. But you two lack consensus on the problem that this solution is supposed to solve, so he won't cooperate with the solution. This leads you to think he doesn't care about the problem—that is, about you.

"So let's start with this: Rachel, what exactly is it that Jackson does or doesn't do regarding sex that upsets you? You never know—we might be able to address your pain about various things without requiring that he stop watching porn."

They both eyed me warily, as if I were conning them out of something, although they couldn't figure out exactly what. "If you're wondering what I'm pulling here, I'll tell you: You've been fighting about the wrong thing, so no matter what solution one of you proposes, the other rejects it and you make zero progress. I want to get you out of that dead end by finding one or more problems you can agree you want to fix. Then you can choose to work as a team to resolve them." They seemed startled by my directness. But I was staying a step ahead of them, which they liked. So we proceeded.

They found it difficult to talk about themselves without blaming each other. It was pretty standard stuff: he makes me feel insecure; she doesn't turn me on; you don't really desire me; you don't tell me what you're thinking; and so on. So over and over, I gently interrupted, reframing their complaints as self-disclosures: I feel insecure; I don't turn myself on with you; I don't feel desired; I don't know what you're thinking, and I'd love to. Little by little we defined the experiences they were having with each other.

"OK, I'll tell you how I feel," Rachel eventually said to Jackson. "I'm afraid you don't want to have sex with me because I don't look like a porn actress, and that when we do finally have sex you're thinking of them instead of me."

Brava—perfectly said. Sad, but perfectly said.

And Jackson was able to get it: "Doc, I guess this is where I sympathize instead of telling her she's wrong, right?" Bravo—perfectly done. "Rachel, that sounds lousy. I'm sorry you feel that way," he said.

They both looked at me—now what?

"Jackson, if you don't want Rachel to feel that way, how would you like her to feel?" "Um, I think she's pretty attractive, so I'd like her to feel that way. And I know we don't have sex very much, but when we do, I'd like her to know I'm focused on her."

"Thanks, but I don't get that," Rachel said testily. "If you're used to gorgeous bodies and deep-throating, why come to me? And when you do, why focus on me instead of fantasizing about some fabulous babe?"

This is where things get interesting—when people finally start talking honestly. Sometimes I think patients need me to speak for them, and I do. Other times I feel I can trust a patient to speak the truth gracefully and without rancor. So I turned to Jackson, took a quiet breath, and motioned for him to answer her.

"Honey, it's not real," he said. "True, I get excited and have nice big orgasms when I jack off to porn. But they're videos, not people. They don't kiss me, don't hug me, don't know my name. It's true that your body isn't like an actress's body, but you're real. I can think about them when I'm alone. When I'm with you—especially if we're getting along—I want to focus on you. On us."

"But look at this body," she said tearily. "My hair's turning gray, my butt's getting bigger, and my boobs sag. I know you love nice boobs. I just don't have them anymore. So with unlimited porn babes to look at and think about, how can you get excited with me? Why would you want to?"

"Wait a minute," I jumped in. "First of all," I said, looking at her warmly, "at your age breasts don't sag, they relax." They laughed, and the mood lightened a bit. "Second, that's your work right now, Rachel—to imagine your body as an attractive sexual object to Jackson, to imagine that you bring something to him that he can process into erotic feelings. Every adult has to start doing that work sooner or later. And don't tell me it's easier with men. As they get older, men have to envision themselves as being sexually attractive and competent, too—and it's not always easy."

"I don't know," said Rachel quietly. "Well," I said, "as long as you can't imagine yourself as attractive in Jackson's eyes, you'll always be suspicious about his experience with you, and you'll never be able to enjoy it yourself. This isn't a porn problem," I said. "And getting him to stop watching porn won't fix this problem."

"Maybe this is related," she said thoughtfully. "I think I'm nervous about how successful he's getting. It's not like I think he'll leave me," she said, "but that he's going off on new adventures without me, and that I'll be boring compared to all the exciting new people he's meeting." "That sounds scary," said Jackson right on cue. We both looked at him and chuckled.

I leaned in her direction. "So your kids are growing up, your husband is growing up, and you're imagining feeling left behind by everyone?" At that she burst into tears. And that issue—supporting our loved ones' autonomy even while we fear abandonment—was a key to the entire case.

When Rachel saw that his porn-watching wasn't the problem, she told him he could go ahead and watch—"as long as you connect with me on a regular basis." Pleased to have part of his adulthood back, Jackson agreed—"as long as you're usually nice to me." I clarified this—"*usually* nice, not *always* nice—right?" He smiled and agreed that that's what he meant.

Jackson had to change his thinking a bit, and point himself more in her direction when thoughts of sex crossed his mind. This didn't mean he'd abandon masturbating to porn altogether, just that he'd remind himself of options with her—and, presumably, choose sex with her more frequently.

That is, in fact, the way it worked out. They still had to navigate their family situation, in which he worked too hard, spent less time with his kids than he (or she, or they) wished, and she struggled to create a satisfying life outside her role as homemaker. But they did it with more affection and trust than they had in years. They even had a little more sex, which led to more smiles. Which sometimes led to a little more sex.

Case B

JOHN & BORA: THE MAN WHO TRIED TO COMMUNICATE THROUGH PORN

Although John worked for a well-known high-tech company, he was not an engineer—he was a designer. Unlike many of my more science-oriented patients, he has friends outside work, listens to music, can talk about the news, and cares if his clothes match. Our session was often a change of pace for me in the day's routine of computer geniuses.

Ironically, it was John's non-tech wife Bora who was inhibited and non-social. Bora felt especially self-conscious about sex. The daughter of small-town Korean immigrants, she always felt inferior to American women. They all seemed so self-confident and energetic to her. Sex had never been mentioned during her childhood, and like many Korean women she was completely unprepared for a sexually dynamic marriage—which is what her artistic American husband had envisioned for them.

John and Bora came to therapy because he wanted her to watch porn with him as a preliminary to sex, and she was extremely uncomfortable doing so. Meanwhile, their sex life was languishing. He was upset. So was she—mostly because he was upset, which meant she was failing as a wife. His response was to urge her to watch a variety of porn with him, and he was confused by her lack of interest, no matter what kind he suggested.

"Bora, why does John want you to watch porn together?" I asked. He started to answer, but I interrupted. In a respectful tone, she replied, "Perhaps you could ask him." "No, I'd like you to answer," I responded gently. This is a common approach I use to find out what people know (or imagine) about their mate's thinking and expectations. "I don't know," she said quietly, an answer that would be common from her in the weeks to come. "I think he wants me to imitate the girls in the videos?"

John almost jumped out of his chair like an impatient third-grader dying to give the right answer. But I stopped him, saying, "Let's let her continue." "Bora," I asked, "I don't know if John wants you to imitate the girls in the videos, but if he does—*if* he does—why would he want that?" John wanted to answer again, but again I gently refused to let him.

"To get me to be good in sex," said Bora quietly. "So far I know I'm not, and he's disappointed." Ah, now we were getting somewhere.

John, of course, was bursting to speak. "No, no, no," he said emotionally. "That's not it. I want to help you get really excited so you can desire and enjoy our lovemaking. I'm looking for the right porn to get you aroused with me." Turning to me, he said, "Doc, tell her there are many kinds of porn, and that she should give me a chance to find the right one."

For her part, Bora wanted to satisfy her husband. But the more exotic the videos he shared, the more confused and pessimistic she became. If those videos are his idea of a good sexual experience, she reasoned, "I'm never going to please him," she said sadly. "I'm not like those girls," she told him, "and it seems you want sex things that . . . that . . . well, I don't know how you find a girl like that, but I'm not one of them."

Given the videos John tried to share with her, Bora had gradually become convinced that his taste in sex ran extreme—threesomes, climaxing on a woman's face, rough fellatio, sex in public. To avoid feeling pressured to do stuff she didn't want to do, or to continually turn him down (and to maintain her dignity), Bora's response over time was to quietly withdraw from sex.

I didn't want them damaging their relationship any further. "I suggest four weeks off from genital sex," I said to their surprise at the end of our session. "Is that OK? If you want to kiss or hug or cuddle, go right ahead," I said, "but do it knowing that it won't lead to sex, OK? You can each masturbate privately if you like, but no sex with each other. Agreed?" They agreed—she with relief, he with curiosity.

When they returned two weeks later, they had indeed refrained from sex. And they were more physically affectionate. I asked them why, and Bora reported feeling freer, less self-critical, closer to him, and less anxious. I smiled. "Interesting, don't you think?" We talked about other aspects of our previous session. They agreed it had been valuable, encouraging them to talk about "intimacy." "You mean sex?" I asked gently. Yes, of course.

"Maybe you two don't have a porn problem," I soon continued. "Porn is sort of the way you communicate about sex," I said, "and it's not very efficient. It's confusing things rather than clarifying them." OK, I had their attention. So what did I think was their problem?

Although they loved each other, John and Bora hadn't expressed their sexual interests to each other clearly enough, and so each had incomplete information about the other. Each had to fill in the missing pieces by imagining stories about each other—stories that made things more complicated, not less. And this had been going on for several years.

Bora thought John wanted to know exactly what sexual activities she wanted, but her vocabulary (and comfort) for that conversation was quite limited. She knew how she wanted to feel, but he didn't seem to be asking about that—and she didn't want to make things worse by talking about vague things like her feelings.

John wanted hot sex, but Bora seemed uninterested. And he couldn't get her to talk about her interests in a way he found helpful. He believed he simply needed to figure out what intense things she would like, and then they'd do them, and live happily (and hotly) ever after. So he thought they just needed to go through the catalog of stereotyped human eroticism contained in porn, hoping she'd eventually see things she wanted. Too much the eager administrator, he made only limited attempts to get her input, which wasn't nearly enough for her.

It was both charming and heartbreaking to see these two people who, most of all, wanted the other to be sexually satisfied—but somehow couldn't make it happen.

"John," I asked, "what message do you think Bora's getting from your porn-of-the-week approach?" He hadn't really thought about it. "Do you think she's feeling more relaxed, more self-accepting, more curious about her body? Do you think she's feeling more loved?"

He realized that she probably didn't. "The porn's not helping, is it?" he said slowly. "And Bora," I asked, "can you imagine that John might be using porn as a way of trying to understand your sexuality better? You might think that's an odd way to do it, but can you imagine that might be what he's doing?"

Bora turned to him with a simple and direct question: "Is it?" When he nodded and said it was, the room was quiet for a long time. There was no reason for me to insert myself into their delicate dance of discovery at this point. Finally, Bora spoke.

"My husband," she said with a warm smile, "we don't need those ladies to help us understand each other. Come home and talk to me."

He did.

They only needed a few more sessions after that, which were entirely different. I helped them talk; brokered a few agreements; challenged a couple of myths they both believed (like a real man could make a woman climax from intercourse, if she were a real woman); laid out some facts about contraception, lubricants, and sex toys; and rather than teach them sexual anatomy, encouraged them to teach each other about their bodies.

Later, at our final session, I asked about porn. "Still not for me," Bora said simply. "It's for John. But privately. And not when we both want sex!" Which, apparently, they were starting to enjoy regularly.

Case C

JEVON: THE MAN WHO TRIED TO ORGANIZE THE INTERNET

"He's a nice guy with a massive porn problem," said the voicemail. "Maybe the biggest one that even you've ever seen." It was a message from a local therapist who had just referred me a case.

And so Jevon called me that evening. He said that he had been seeing this therapist about two months, and that when he told her about his porn stash, she replied, "Well, that's beyond what I know about. You should see Dr. Marty Klein." We made an appointment for later that month.

Jevon seemed like a nice guy, a supervisor in a local post office branch. When I met him he was still wearing the blue-gray tie he wore all day at work—unusual in sartorially informal Silicon Valley. In a friendly but straightforward way, he sat down and got right to the point.

"My therapist said I should see you. I think she's a little freaked out by my porn collection. We've been getting along fine—she's very good—but two weeks ago I mentioned relaxing with my collection, and she asked a few questions, and when I told her what I had, she looked nervous and said, 'Um, this is a bit beyond my training. You better see a sex therapist,' and you were one of two people she recommended. You were the first one who returned my call, so here we are."

"Two- or three-minute snippets of adult films," he said. "Extracts from longer movies."

He had about 50,000 of them—yes, about 50,000. That's a lot of *anything*. I said, "I'm mandated to report anyone owning images of adult-child sexuality." "Oh, there's no child porn in it," he said. "I don't go for that stuff. I know some guys do, but not me. I like good old-fashioned naked ladies and regular sex, that's all I have." He seemed pretty definite about it. So with that issue out of the way, we could proceed.

As matter-of-factly as I could, I asked lots of questions, and Jevon answered them all. Yes, the videos showed a pretty wide range of activities. No, most didn't involve a lot of kissing scenes. Yes, he was still acquiring new ones. No, he never looked at the whole collection all at once—at most, just a section of the collection once in a while. No, he rarely masturbated to the videos already in his collection—it was always to new videos.

So what was his vision in assembling and expanding this collection? Not surprisingly, his answer was quite mundane: "Nothing, really. It just seemed like a good idea. Fun. Relaxing. I never imagined it would get so big, but it did."

It started about six years ago when his wife went to Phoenix to care for her ailing mother for about a month. He'd go to the Internet to find porn with which to masturbate. He used a common free site that had thumbnails (little freeze-frame pictures) of videos; click on the thumbnail and up pops your video. They were organized by category—romantic, threesome, gay, older women, etc. Very convenient, perfect for the modern consumer.

He'd pick a category ("I like woman–woman or woman–woman–man," he said), click on a thumbnail, watch, and begin masturbating. "But then I'd start thinking, 'Well, what about all the other videos?' So I'd switch to another, and the same thing would happen, so I'd switch from one to the next to the next about 30, 40 times in a single session of masturbation," he said.

"Sounds a little hectic," I said sympathetically.

"Yes, and it meant one hand was always on the mouse," he said. "Sometimes it was hard to maintain the continuous arousal that a person wants during masturbation. The different videos didn't always match up in intensity—one might be from a foreplay scene, another showing people really going at it, etc., so sometimes it was a little weird.

"Anyway," he continued, "I started feeling that I was missing more videos than I was watching—which of course I am, when you think about it. So I just got into finding videos I thought I might like to watch in the future, and saving them in files inside my computer. And I categorized them just like on the porn website—pregnant women, or Russian models, or drunk women getting gang-banged, or whatever."

So did he find the activity of locating and storing images sexually arousing? "Hmm, interesting question," he said. "Well, in the first few months, I'd be erect most of the time that I was doing it," he said. "In fact, sometimes I'd stop and jack off, and after I climaxed, that would be the end of finding and sorting for the night," he recalled ruefully. "But now I don't get quite so excited, so it's easier to keep building the collection, I don't get so distracted, and I can focus."

So he was quite surprised when his wife accused him of being a porn addict. "She knew I used porn for years, and never said a word," he said. "We had friends, we had family, we had church, there was nothing wrong." Then she got laid off from her job, and their financial situation became precarious. "And ever since," he says now, "she gives me a bad time about it. I don't know why. I just know that I have this harmless hobby, my wife says I'm a porn addict, and I say she should leave me alone to do my thing. She's mad, I'm mad, and I think somehow the church, or recovery group, or whomever, is giving her bad advice."

And indeed, she had been told that he was "addicted," "disrespectful to her and all women," and "borderline unfaithful," and that he should just give up porn and accept her as his only mate. Jevon was confused: "All that stuff isn't true, is it? I thought what I was doing was harmless. Now it turns out it isn't? Is there something wrong with me?"

"Jevon," I said, "you've accumulated 50,000 of something. Forget what the something is for a second. Fifty thousand of anything is a lot, isn't it?" "I guess so," he nodded. "You guess so? Listen, don't just agree with me to be polite. If you don't realize that 50,000 toy cars or 50,000 bars of hotel soap or 50,000 books about knitting or 50,000 baseball cards is a lot of those things, just say so."

"OK, OK, I get it—I have an unusual situation here." "Yes!" I said, "You've created an unusual situation, which you maintain every week. Right?" "Right," he said, sounding like he was starting to understand. "So Jevon, we have to figure out what this means, right?" "Yeah, Doc, I get your point. Maybe collecting 50,000 thumbnails is about something other than the thumbnails themselves?" "Exactly," I said with a smile.

After a few sessions, I learned more about Jevon's journey. He had already spoken to his minister, his physician, and his brother-in-law. They all told him he had a porn problem, and that he had to give it up. He had tried this approach on several occasions, but he couldn't bring himself to destroy his carefully assembled collection, and whenever he tried to stop masturbating to porn, he'd eventually "fall off the wagon," as he put it. Jevon ruefully took this as evidence that there was indeed something wrong with him, even though he couldn't figure out what. After all, his hobby wasn't really hurting anyone, was it?

So his epiphany with me—this his collecting 50,000 porn thumbnails might be about something other than the porn thumbnails—was a novel approach to his mystery, which no one had suggested. That's the problem with living in a PornPanic: People get distracted by the porn aspect of a situation and have trouble seeing any other part of it.

So Jevon and I talked and talked. We talked about women, about sex, about porn, and about lots of other things.

I found out he wasn't having very much sex with his wife, about which he felt quite sad. She was disappointed that he hadn't gone further up the ranks of the postal service, and she often expressed her resentment about this, comparing him to his more financially successful brothers. Jevon and his wife only shared physical affection on a sporadic basis, and he was always feeling emotionally hungry—or anxiously awaiting the next abrupt loss of emotional nourishment.

He had almost no friends on the job, because people didn't feel comfortable socializing with the boss, and there was really no one at his supervisory level.

One day I asked him to give his porn thumbnail collection a name. After about ten seconds he named it The Gang. Why? "Because they're always there for me, and with them I'm comfortable; I have a familiar feeling, like I belong."

I wrote down Jevon's words, and then read them back to him. His face flushed, he looked down for a long time, and then he faced me, slowly shaking his head. "What kind of man says that?" he asked. "Am I really keeping a huge collection of naked ladies on video so I have a place where I can relax and feel like I belong?"

His eyes showed grief as he shook his head. We continued the following week.

"The question of you masturbating and the question of The Gang are two separate things," I said after we settled in and briefly discussed his week. "There are plenty of other ways to masturbate. How you relate to The Gang is a much bigger question, isn't it?"

"I guess so," he said. "I guess getting rid of the collection doesn't mean I can't relax or masturbate in other ways." "Right," I said, "although getting rid of the collection presumably means not building another one, right?" "Oh," said Jevon, "I hadn't thought about that." Unconsciously, he had automatically assumed he'd just start another one—build another gang. "That really shows that there's something more going on here than just thumbnails, doesn't it," he asked glumly. Of course he was right—a great insight.

He didn't really have a porn problem; he had a problem he was expressing through porn. Everyone knows this common dynamic—people abandoning their families for golf don't really have a golf problem; people forgetting their mother-in-law's birthday every year don't really have a memory problem. But when the vehicle for expressing a problem is porn, somehow people forget this and assume the person has a porn problem.

There was nothing wrong with Jevon's reality testing—he knew the whole thing was a fantasy, a game he played with himself, using videos as playing pieces. It just so happened that the videos showed explicit sex, instead of famous home runs or horse races. Regardless, "the thought of doing without my Gang, I dunno, it's a little scary," he said more than once.

So we had solved the mystery of the massive porn collection. Now we could discuss things that really mattered—like how he was going to say goodbye to The Gang and how he could get more intimacy in his life.

He needed to talk with his wife.

They needed to reconnect, which meant they each needed to reveal their needs and their disappointments at letting their relationship go. I suggested couples counseling, but Jevon thought his wife would be skeptical. "As long as you two talk, and talk meaningfully, it doesn't matter how you do it," I said. "A therapist, a pastor, long walks in the park, face-to-face in the kitchen—as long as you talk." He agreed.

So they talked. Apparently, it was pretty rough. They talked more. They discussed separating. They decided against it. Jevon went on an antidepressant, which helped him open up to her a little more. He talked about how he needed affection, how a few kind words from her meant the world to him. She was surprised—she didn't think he needed much from her, and she thought sex was at the top of his list. When she found out how lonely he felt, her heart melted.

He decided to masturbate less, to consciously turn toward his wife when he wanted comfort or connection. They resumed having sex a little. The antidepressant, plus his own fear of failure, made that complicated, too. But they stuck with it, and the sex slowly improved.

Jevon was still nervous about facing life without The Gang. But he had made some significant steps and was on his way.

Chapter Seven

HOW DOES PORN
AFFECT CONSUMERS?

Every good citizen should be concerned about any consumer product whose use inevitably leads to violence, mental illness, and community dysfunction—which anti-porn activists assert about pornography.

Sociology professor Ronald Weitzer of George Washington University has identified a particular theoretical approach to prostitution and pornography—the Oppression Paradigm. "This perspective," he says, "depicts all types of sex work and pornography as exploitative, violent, and perpetuating gender inequality. This paradigm does not hold that exploitation and violence are variables"—present or absent in varying degrees—"but are instead constants central to the very definition of prostitution, pornography, and stripping."[1]

As we'll see here in the words of many anti-porn activists, this approach "substitutes ideology for rigorous empirical analysis."[2] It's a key part of the cultural shift from porn as a problem of immorality to porn as a problem of public health and danger. In other words, it's a key aspect of today's PornPanic.

As Eithne Johnson says, "Feminist anti-porn presentations [at colleges and activist events] rely on an understanding of pornography as 'patriarchal propaganda for violence against women' and on women's victim status . . . They appear to have been designed to shock and frighten the audience through the use of slide shows depicting violent and highly atypical imagery."[3] In this way, anti-porn educators "teach" audiences how to "properly" perceive porn's "real" messages.

From all the anguish, claims, and demands for the abolition of pornography over the past 40 years, one would think there was ample evidence demonstrating the individual and social harms of consuming pornography. Political and religious movements devoted to eliminating pornography often claim to be based on fact, vaguely noting that "Research shows" or "Mounting evidence makes clear. . . ."[4]

A typical example is Robert Jensen, who dismisses empirical research, preferring anecdotes "instead of being paralyzed by the limitations of social science."[5] Susan Brownmiller rejects science as unnecessary altogether: "Does one need scientific methodology in order to conclude that the anti-female propaganda that permeates our nation's cultural output promotes a climate in which acts of sexual hostility directed against women are not only tolerated but ideologically encouraged?"[6]

If you're going to try to regulate the private behavior of 50 million people, the answer is simple: Yes.

Is there any evidence that consuming pornography is actually dangerous? President Lyndon Johnson's commission looked but couldn't find any evidence. President Richard Nixon's commission looked but couldn't find it. And the Meese Commission—specifically chartered by President Ronald Reagan in 1986 to prove porn dangerous—couldn't find it, either. The report stated its *belief* that porn is dangerous, but admitted they could find no evidence to prove it. Three presidential commissions. No evidence—they each explicitly said so.

The Canadian government's report? Same "reluctant" conclusion: insufficient evidence that porn is dangerous. The British government's report? No empirical data to link pornography and harm.

Since the 1970s, activists like Susan Brownmiller and Robin Morgan have confidently stated that pornography "degraded" and actually harmed women, with no evidence whatsoever. Since then, a chorus of feminists, religious conservatives, politicians, and anti-sex work activists has repeated this alleged truth so frequently that the public thinks it's true. And like the legendary Holy Grail that fervent believers have pursued for a thousand years, they claim that this precious, wondrous thing—data showing porn's dangers—surely exists.

Because without this proof, all that people like Andrea Dworkin, Catharine MacKinnon, Donna Rice Hughes, John Stoltenberg, and Pamela Paul have is their anger and their mistrust of sexuality, or men, or both. Without it, they quote Dear Abby and Oprah, a handful of old, discredited studies, an increase in plastic surgery and anal sex, and the self-serving anecdotes of the "porn addiction" industry.

As if wishing could make it so, they make enough noise to create the illusion that real data exist. Besides, they face no intellectual competition from the media, political class, the therapy profession, or any other part of society. In today's porn-prejudiced world, how many reasonable men are going to stand up and say, "I use porn and it hasn't affected me?" How many women will stand up and say, "My husband uses porn and it doesn't hurt us?" How many dentists, junior high school teachers, city councilmembers, janitors, soccer coaches, church board members, and marriage counselors who use porn will stand up and say, "I've used porn for years and plan to continue?"

Anti-porn activists are so attached to their ideology that they persevere despite the lack of data. When society-level research couldn't support their conclusion, they turned to ongoing investigations on the individual level. Still cited today by anti-porn activists, these projects gave undergraduates a narrow set of attitudinal choices after showing them pornography and concluded that porn influenced the guys' attitudes about rape.[7]

But no one has been able to replicate these troubling results—in fact, when given open-ended choices, subsequent lab subjects related to women far more gently than in the original study.[8]

And no one has shown that rape-tolerating attitudes expressed in a lab by college students lead to an increase in actual rape in the real world anyway. According to the U.S. Department of Justice, American colleges, where rates of porn use are extraordinarily *high,* have *lower* rates of sexual violence than comparable communities elsewhere in America.[9] Nevertheless, activist Gail Dines still passionately claims that, "Porn tells men that they have no sexual boundaries, morality, or compassion for women. It strips them of their humanity."[10] Jensen adds—without any data whatsoever—that "pornography demands that men abandon empathy" for women and for female performers.[11]

So what is a good citizen to conclude?

There simply is no public health crisis caused by the widespread consumption of pornography. There is, rather, a long-term, one-sided propaganda war.

Today there's talk of America's "rape culture," and how our society has to acknowledge and challenge it, using every tool including eliminating porn and eliminating rape jokes.[12] "America's rape culture" seems to be the preface to every conversation condemning pornography.

But here's a fact systematically ignored by rape activists and the mass media: While there's still too damn much rape, the rate of rape has gone *down* since Internet porn flooded America's homes. Documented by the government, reported in places such as the *Journal of Sex Research,* the University of Hawaii's Pacific Center for Sex and Society, and Northwestern University Law School,[13] the rate of rape in the United States has steadily declined since the explosion of Internet porn. (Yes, rape is underreported—now, as it has been every year.[14])

So how can activists claim that porn viewing leads to rape and other awful consequences? Only by ignoring the facts. And so Morality in Media (recently rebranded as the National Center on Sexual Exploitation) and other groups point obsessively to "violent porn"—a media product showing pretend behavior—and claim it's responsible for sexual violence in the real world. They never tell the truth about the decline in the rate of sexual violence. That wouldn't be a very good fundraising tool. Besides, activist Dines says the science doesn't matter. She "knows" there's a connection: "At the core of contemporary pornography is contempt for women. One need not look at the most violent or sadomasochistic pornography to reach this conclusion."[15] Of course that's all she ever shows or discusses.

Anti-porn activists are right about one thing, of course—there is some vicious, sadistic porn available (although they dramatically overestimate how much there is, and how popular it is). Some of us wonder how anyone can maintain an erection while watching it (and indeed, very few people do watch it). But how does this affect the viewer of such material when he walks out of his house? Depending on which science you look at, the answer is either "mostly not" or "not at all." Let's look at what the two most respected names in the field say.

UCLA researcher Neil Malamuth posits a Confluence model, in which pornography is like alcohol: Its effects depend on the person (and to a lesser extent, the cultural context). He notes that for most people, moderate use of either one leads to relaxation. But for a few people, moderate use is difficult to maintain, and too much use can lead to disaster. So what are the risk factors that identify men who are vulnerable to negative outcomes of high porn use?

a. Hostile masculinity, expressed as narcissism, attitudes accepting violence against women, and sexual arousal to violence or power over women;
b. Impersonal orientation to sexuality, a result of growing up with high parental conflict, physical or emotional abuse, and anti-social features in adolescence

Men with both of these constellations are more likely to engage in sexual violence (of course, "more likely" is still an extremely small number). According to Malamuth, porn affects this high-risk group differently than other men, and violent porn affects them even more strongly.[16] "Pornography use can be a risk factor of sexually aggressive outcomes, principally for men who are high on other risk factors and who use pornography frequently," he says.[17]

After reviewing a range of data and possible theories to explain them, researchers at Toronto's Centre for Addiction and Mental Health essentially agreed with this conclusion, without taking a position on exactly who would be most vulnerable to the effects of high levels of violent pornography:

"From the existing evidence, we argue that individuals who are already predisposed to sexually offend are the most likely to show an effect of pornography exposure and are the most likely to show the strongest effects. Men who are not predisposed are unlikely to show an effect; if there actually is an effect, it is likely to be transient because these men would not normally seek violent pornography.

"Overall," they conclude, "there is little support for a direct causal link between pornography use and sexual aggression."[18]

Veteran Canadian sex researcher William Fisher recognizes the value of Malamuth's work, but feels it leaves too many questions unanswered—and overlooks some of its own assumptions. For example, Fisher says that an individual man's sex drive is a key variable: that it is correlated positively with use of porn, with use of aggressive porn, and with sexual aggression.

Fisher also believes that what some psychologists call "attachment style" influences both men's and women's emotional experience of pornography. Interestingly, when Fisher repeated Donnerstein's lab studies (which essentially found that undergraduate men who looked at violent porn then had harsher attitudes toward women), he gave subjects an additional option—to *speak* with the women afterwards. Fisher reports that most men did so, and then did *not* show the increase in violent attitudes toward women that Donnerstein found.[19]

So **the scientific evidence is consistent on one fact: Watching nonviolent porn, or viewing violent porn only occasionally, doesn't encourage sexually violent behavior** in the real world. You will virtually never hear about this scientific consensus from PornPanic activists.

However, the evidence does suggest two different possibilities. Either:

1. *Some* men are at higher risk for sexually violent behavior if they watch a *lot* of *violent* porn (which, contrary to Dines' claim, you have to seek out if you want to view it),

   or

2. Watching a lot of violent porn does not increase one's risk for sexually violent behavior.

Note that "at higher risk" is *not* the same as "leads to." There isn't a *scientist* alive who claims that someone sits around minding his own business, watches some porn (violent or otherwise), and suddenly decides to get up and rape somebody. And yet that fiction is exactly what many anti-porn activists want you to believe.

Of course, people who choose to watch a lot of violent porn are not a random sample of Americans. People who choose that form of entertainment may have atypical hormonal issues, personality structures, relationship styles, substance abuse, previous experiences, or other ongoing issues that make them more likely to engage in sexually aggressive behavior. Indeed, reports of search terms by porn consumers almost never show words like "violence," "harm," "pain," or "degradation" among the most popular terms.

In the real world, a very large percentage of adult American men (up to half) look at porn; a very, very, very small percentage of adult men watch a lot of violent porn; and a tiny percentage of adult men engage in sexually violent behavior.

WHAT IS THE "VIOLENCE" IN "VIOLENT PORNOGRAPHY"?

If we're going to talk about "violent porn," we need a vocabulary and some data.

Rebecca Whisnant, for example, claims that in most porn, "hostile and humiliating acts against women are commonplace," and that "aggression against women is the rule rather than the exception."[20] If true, this assertion is of great importance—but she offers no evidence. Similarly, Dines says that "body-punishing" sex is now the norm, harming actresses every day[21]— despite an almost total lack of complaints by actresses themselves.

Periodically, an item in the news (or someone running for re-election) encourages another assessment of "violence on television." Estimates of its occurrence always vary wildly, depending on how "violence" is defined: news shows? War movies? *CSI*? Documentaries? Westerns? Horror films? *Gone With the Wind*? *Ghostbusters*? It's an interesting call—and the *definition* of "violence" is the primary determinant in how much violence studies have found.

The same is true with measuring "violent porn" (and porn that's "demeaning to women"), which according to activists is the most common kind. Consider these activities commonly depicted in porn:

Two women and one man having sex together
Two men and one woman having sex together
A woman masturbating while someone observes
A woman involved in fellatio while on her knees, her back, standing, or sitting
Intercourse with the woman on her hands and knees, entered from behind
Cunnilingus (and yes, a woman has to spread her legs and expose her vulva to facilitate this)
A woman shown with partially or completely shaved or waxed pubic area
Anal sex (male penis or finger or female finger, female anus)
Spanking (man spanks woman or woman spanks man)
A man stimulating a woman vaginally with a dildo or vibrator

A man stimulating a woman anally with a dildo or vibrator
A woman tied up and enjoying sex with several men
Sex between older man and younger (over 18) woman
Older woman seduces younger (over 18) woman or man
Man ejaculating on woman's body or face, with her encouragement
Man bending woman's legs way back as he slides his penis into her vagina
    while she's on her back

Which of these should be coded as "violence"? Various anti-porn activists say most or all of them. Virtually all porn consumers would say none. Certainly, 100 percent of people who do these things consensually in real life would say none. Hence the wildly different estimates of how much "violent porn" and "porn demeaning to women" there is. (And again, scientific evidence suggests that the behavioral impacts of watching so-called violent porn on most men is negligible.)

To put it another way, someone's opinion about what's violent or demeaning in porn says more about their concepts of sexuality than it does about the porn they're describing. And because so many women enjoy these activities in real life, the opinion that these activities are demeaning or violent is hardly universal. Women (or men) who don't like some or all of these activities shouldn't do them—but no one can say that they're inherently violent or demeaning to *all* women.

We should be troubled by any analysis insisting that the portrayal of consenting fellatio or masturbating for a lover (to select just two common acts from the list) is inherently demeaning.

Finally, let's remember that many adults play sex games. Pretending to pressure a lover to do what you both enjoy (while he or she pretends to resist) is probably the most common one (it's called teasing). So are biting, hair-pulling, or holding someone down. When consenting people do these things they aren't violence or disrespect, whether at home or on the screen.

Indeed, Professor of Psychology Ana Bridges—no fan of porn—found extreme violence to be rare or non-existent in her sample of 50 top-selling porn videos, whereas "more mild and playful" acts (pinching, biting, slapping, spanking, hair-pulling) were more common. She coded the majority of these as consensual, but nevertheless is concerned they might send the message that people enjoy such things—as if she needs to protect people from their own sense of enjoyment if it differs from hers.[22]

Ironically, research by Meagan Tyler—who was specifically looking for violence against women in pornography—found a similar result. Examining 98 Editor's Choice Reviews in *Adult Video News*, she found three-quarters contained no violence, and that *none* involved torture, weapons, kicking, attempted murder, or dismemberment—depictions that anti-porn activists say are common. Astonishingly, Tyler contradicts her own data, concluding that "extreme and violent pornography is permeating the industry."[23]

To know if porn is *depicting* a consensual sex game or a character coercing another character, you'd have to watch enough of the film to get the context. Anti-porn activists generally don't. You'd have to ask the director and actors what scene they think they're playing. Anti-porn activists generally don't. Apparently, some don't even care: R.E. Funk believes all penetration is a form of violence,[24] while Jensen condemns depictions of "unusual" sex acts like anal sex and facial ejaculations regardless of consent or female enjoyment. Jensen even condemns sexual acts that are "uncomfortable" or leave a woman sore[25] (oops, there goes the honeymoon).

* * *

What exactly is the problem with depicting coercion for a viewer's entertainment? Everyone agrees that most adults enjoy films and TV shows that depict coercion and violence on a regular basis. World theatre, cinema, and literature (including the Bible) have portrayed such themes since these respective media began—because these are important and entertaining themes for humans to engage.

Every culture also features sporting events that are dangerous for participants and that attract large crowds of spectators. In our own era, sports including NASCAR, ice hockey, football, boxing, MMA, rugby, motocross, and bull-riding attract spectators specifically there to witness violence, injury, and occasionally death. This is also true for those attending spectacles like cockfighting, dogfighting, and Pamplona's bull-running. And, of course, many of television's most popular shows are violent.

Activists who don't like the reality that many people enjoy watching such material should blame the wiring of the human nervous system, not pornography.

Here's a final inconvenient truth: millions of healthy men and women (gay, straight, and bisexual) like to *pretend* they're involved with violence, coercion, force, and aggression when they make love in real life. Are we not allowed to watch portrayals of these *pretend* experiences in porn?

To repeat: The rate of rape has gone down as the availability of porn has gone up. That effect has also been documented in Germany, Denmark, Sweden, Croatia, China, Czech Republic, and Japan.[26] Whether or not Americans live in a "rape culture," whether that culture is being increasingly glorified or pornified, there is no epidemic of actual sexual violence since free porn flooded America's homes, universities, and offices.

Instead of blaming porn for a non-existent epidemic, people should be wondering what we can learn from the good news about the recent decade-long *decrease* in the rate of sexual assault.

WHAT DO PORN CONSUMERS SAY?

Debates about the effect of porn on consumers are almost always missing something: the voices of porn consumers themselves. Given contemporary sensitivities about excluding any voices from cultural discussions, this omission of porn consumers' voices is both notable and meaningful.

As a result, porn consumers in public policy discussion exist only in stereotype—variously lonely, horny, secretive, addicted, beauty-obsessed, compulsively masturbating, aggressive, selfish, alienated from their partner if they have one, and from social reality if they don't. The "porn consumer" has joined other stereotypical sexual characters who may not speak for themselves, such as the pedophile, the fetishist, and the curious child.

Sociologist Alan McKee says "there is a systematic 'othering' of pornography consumers in academic research and in public debate about the genre. They cannot know themselves; they cannot speak for themselves; they must be represented."[27] Psychologist Feona Attwood notes society does this "as part of more extensive programmes of myth-making about sex and technology."[28]

Like the stereotyped and publicly "othered" gay community of 30 or 40 years ago, porn consumers are continually culturally disappeared, as if they aren't thoughtful parents, caring spouses, or selective media consumers, and as if their reactions to porn are simple and monolithic, and that porn has the same functions at all times for all audiences, regardless of age, class, relationship status, etc.

According to many studies, porn users often say that porn enhances their real-life sexual relationships; in several studies users—and their partners, by the way—are more likely to report positive relationship impacts of porn than negative ones. These positive impacts include improved attitude toward sexuality, greater variety of sexual behaviors, and improved quality of life.[29]

Not surprisingly, many studies show that porn consumption does *not* appear to be linked to negative attitudes toward women.[30] For the most part, porn shows women enjoying sex and pleasing their partners. Why would we assume viewers of such scenes would feel worse about women?

Another arena is which porn users' voices are missing regards the question, "Is porn a form of infidelity?" While some women feel it is and others feel it isn't, very few male users think it is. While sincere people may disagree on this question, the public narrative is typically "these selfish men commit adultery via porn, their poor wives are betrayed, and men don't care that they've done this awful thing." This is at great variance from the typical men's narrative; again, why is that voice of experience—which could actually provide emotional comfort to women—disappeared in this way?

Porn users' voices are also conspicuously missing when anyone discusses the common idea that porn use makes men dissatisfied with their partners' bodies, leading to a decline in women's self-esteem. While women's fears are often quoted (and reified by anti-porn activists as an accurate perception of male porn users), the media (and of course activists) almost never check with men themselves about this. Research[31] and my own clinical experience make it clear that few males actually feel that porn use makes them more critical of their partners' bodies. If men's voices were part of the social dialog about this, much female anguish could be soothed. But again, that would challenge the radical narrative—the Oppression Paradigm described previously—that porn use oppresses all women, particularly the partners of users.

If you ask most porn consumers about their porn experience, most would say it's fine—not the centerpiece of life, not their reason for living, merely "fine." They would mostly sound like normal people: If they're in a couple they mostly have affection for their mates. If their mate knows they watch porn, she isn't traumatized by it, nor has she threatened divorce over it. And if their mate is upset about their porn-watching, these average porn consumers are more likely to be regretful than defiant.

In other words, most porn consumers are ordinary people who don't fit the popular consumer-as-selfish-victimizer narrative (or the secondary narrative of being addicted, manipulated victims themselves). And that's why their voices are excluded by anti-porn activists.

Because activists characterize ordinary consumers as using a product that:

- Makes them violent—which most of them are not
- Reflects their selfishness toward women—which most of them are not
- Causes them to reject their partners—which most of them do not
- Proves that they're selfish or weak—which most of them don't feel they are

Unlike cigarette smokers, most porn users are not trying to quit; unlike gamblers, they don't tell people not to start. If they do have personal problems, porn consumers rarely blame them on watching porn (particularly consumers over 30, who have acquired some sexual experience and perspective).

So while real-life, satisfied porn consumers have plenty to say, anti-porn activists aren't interested. Lacking intellectual integrity, activists apparently don't feel obligated to talk with these men—although of course, they continually quote female "victims" of porn use at length. "I have listened to women tell me about being raped and brutalized by men who wanted to re-enact their favorite porn scene," says Dines.[32] One wonders how many such claims she has actually listened to, and why she values these more than scientific data. Nevertheless, note the assumption—that the average guy's "favorite porn scene" involves "rape and brutalization." Is there any doubt that someone who would rape his wife has deeper problems than the porn he watches?

And so on the rare occasions that porn consumers are referenced, they're caricatures—pathetic losers or selfish bastards who care nothing about hurting their poor wives and girlfriends. According to both research[33] and my own 35 years of clinical work, many of these consumers are actually empathic, good guys.

SO WHY HAS SCIENCE IMPACTED THIS DEBATE SO LITTLE?

Why do Americans swallow the most apocalyptic vision of pornography, when they know that their own husbands don't rape anyone, and their own sons are fairly respectful of women (well, no more disrespectful than they are to men, anyway)? What does it mean that people believe that the effects of porn are so much worse than they are?

According to social psychologists at Western University in Ontario, the popular media "report" negative effects of porn that aren't supported by the research they're quoting. Reporting "no effects" or "mixed effects" makes for boring or confusing copy, so they tend to either not report those studies or to oversimplify them. These researchers found the media over-rely on a set of tired assumptions about porn, including the common tropes of "porn addiction"; that watching porn is a form of adultery; and that it harms relationships, intimacy, and health. Note that the first term doesn't exist in the DSM-5 (the diagnostic manual of the mental health profession), the second is merely a personal opinion (often presented as a self-evident fact), and the third is backed by virtually no data.

The public discourse about porn and its effects is not about making women safer, or helping them feel safer. Rather, it's about delegitimizing (1) men's use of porn and (2) women's lust, while encouraging women to feel like disempowered victims. It's also about feathering the nest of activists and activist organizations. It's a conservative response to the fear of technology and change. It exploits the political reality that porn watchers as a consumer group do not and will not control the narrative of their own activity. Because of shame and social opprobrium, the normal political process ("I'm a car owner and I vote!") doesn't work to balance social conflict about this product or its consumers.

Some couples do have problems that appear driven by porn use. Some men push their partner to do sexual acts she does not want to do. Some men push their partner to watch porn when she'd rather not. And some men explicitly compare their partners to porn actresses—usually (though not always) unfavorably.

But these difficulties are not about porn. They're about anger, power issues, and poor communication. They're about a lack of respect or empathy. They also reflect some women's lack of assertiveness in the face of disrespect or self-ishness (puh-leeze—this is *not* "blaming the victim"; it's noticing that some women don't take care of themselves and their needs).

Such conflict is not unusual in couples, and the vehicle is generally some-thing other than porn (like money, in-laws, or parenting). Problems like these can be dealt with productively, especially if people don't get distracted by the porn (or the in-laws or whatever) and keep their mutual goals in mind. If the problem is actually about sex rather than porn, that can be worked out—if people are willing to talk honestly about sex. Unfortunately, not everyone is. And as we've seen, many activists are more invested in the narrative of male sexual exploitation of females than in helping people communicate and get along.

"Polysemicity" is a fancy word for the common phenomenon that the same thing can mean two different things to two different people. For Laura, being a stripper represents a pathetic collapse of self-worth and the loss of her pro-fessional dreams. For Susie, being a stripper is an assertion of self, of control of her own sexuality, and of saving enough money to go to nursing school. Jane can look at stripping and say, "If I were stripping, it would be a horrible experience," but it isn't for Susie. Maria can say, "If I were stripping, it would be a real feat of emotional strength," but it isn't for Laura.

Anti-porn activists insist that everyone's experience of watching porn must be like *theirs* would be. And anti-porn activists insist that every woman's actual experience of the fantasy activities depicted in porn—deep-throat fel-latio, being spanked, a threesome, whatever—must be as awful as they know it would be *for them.* And so Dines can say, "Porn is the most succinct and crisp deliverer of a woman-hating ideology."[34]

What kind of sadistic, unloving world does Dines inhabit? How is it that Rebecca Whisnant sees so much coercion wherever she looks? How is it that such activists meticulously misread the affection, playfulness, exhibitionism, teasing, desire to be dominated, or sheer eroticism that virtually all porn con-sumers see in most pornography?

(See, for example, Loftus's reassuring work on what men see when they watch porn, and that most know it's a fantasy.[35])

In porn, anti-porn critics see women doing things they believe no sane woman would do, so they see coercion, humiliation, and hostility toward women. Critics don't see depictions of women's pleasure as women's pleasure. They see no collaboration. In porn, critics only see men doing things men want to do (have wild sex) while they see women doing things women sup-posedly *don't* want to do (have wild sex).

So of course they only see women servicing men, women as victims, men as coercive. Critics don't see collaboration in sexual scenes. *This dramatically dismisses female sexuality and lust*—and tells women what they should and shouldn't feel.

It's a reminder of the earnest conversations of 1970s feminists, documented in magazines like *Ms.* and *On Our Backs*: Can you be a feminist and like spanking? Can you be a feminist and like to be entered from behind, or to role-play as a naughty school girl?

Radical anti-porn critics apparently need to get out more and meet a wider spectrum of women. And they need to stop fearing female sexuality in all its richness, darkness, and adult power. Sexuality doesn't have to be wholesome to be healthy.

Chapter Eight

IF YOU'RE CONCERNED ABOUT
YOUR INVOLVEMENT WITH PORN

> Just because you watch a ton of porn
> doesn't mean you have a porn problem.
> Although you might.

Just about every week, here's the kind of pain I hear from one guy or another about his porn-watching:

"I watch more than I intend to"
"I feel guilty"
"Sometimes I have trouble telling what's real"
"I feel inadequate compared to porn"
"I'm afraid the stuff I look at is sick"
"I want a partner with a perfect body"
"My girlfriend says I'm as bad as a rapist or trafficker"
"I know she doesn't like me watching porn"
"I feel like a pathetic loser"
"I don't think it's normal for a grown man to masturbate"
"I don't think it's right for a married man to masturbate"
"I hate keeping a secret"
"I'm afraid I'm addicted"

"God must surely hate me"

"She's always telling me I'm a pervert"

"She's says I'm a selfish bastard"

"I'm always looking at women as if they're naked"

"I can't tell anyone about this"

"I've tried quitting porn more than once, but I keep coming back to it"

"I can't seem to create sex like I see in porn, and it's frustrating"

Some of these guys watch 20 minutes a week. Some of these guys watch 20 times a week. They're all ages and backgrounds; some are fabulously wealthy, others are barely paying their bills every month. For some guys I'm the fourth or fifth therapist they've seen; for others, just coming to a therapist once feels like a shameful failure. Many of them are so flooded by emotion they can't think straight about their situation.

Maybe you're one of these guys, or you know someone who is. So let's talk.

The first step in treating anyone is getting a sense of whether they actually have a problem, and if so, what kind of problem it is. Regardless of what someone's distress is about, here's how I generally think about incoming patients:

1. Someone else says you have problem; and/or
2. You're concerned that you might have a problem; and/or
3. You have an actual problem.

It's the same with problems that are supposedly sex problems, or supposedly porn problems:

1. Someone else says you have problem; and/or
2. You're concerned that you might have a problem; and/or
3. You have an actual problem.

Here are the stories of three different men I saw last year. Can you see that they might need completely different treatment approaches?

Here's Isaac:

"My wife hates that I watch porn two or three times a week. Recently she made me take this test from a website, and it says I'm a porn addict. We go to church every few months—you know, mostly for weddings or baptisms, or when my wife's parents are in town—and sure enough, a few weeks ago the pastor was going on about porn, and how it damages men and their families. My brother-in-law goes to AA meetings, and he said that a lot of people have a porn addiction, especially alcoholics. So he says he's swearing off porn. He says it's harder than giving up drinking. So it feels like everyone's leaning on me to see that I have a porn problem. Do you think I do?"

Here's Mario:

"I've watched porn most of my adult life, and I never gave it a second thought—you know, just a harmless, fun thing. Then I noticed most of the stuff I watch these days is about college girls. Still harmless, I guess, but my own daughter is in high school now, and her friends, wow, some of them are gorgeous young women. I worry that looking at porn and then looking at Celia's friends, well, maybe I'm getting a little confused. Is it OK to have those fantasies? Is porn causing me problems, or will it? I'm still interested in my wife, but sometimes I think about other women when we make love. Is that normal?"

Here's Steve:

"I watch porn every night. It's part of my routine—work late, come home, eat, watch Netflix while I check email, and then go to my favorite porn website. The thing is, I figure I'll just watch a little, but it's like I go into a trance, and don't come out for hours. I'm always amazed that I've been 'gone' so long. Sometimes when I'm struggling to get up in the morning after only five or six hours of sleep I tell myself 'no porn tonight' or 'only 20 minutes of porn tonight.' But that never works, it's another two or three hours of porn, way past midnight. And then in the morning I feel really pathetic. It seems I can't watch less, and I certainly can't give it up altogether. What's wrong with me?"

Very different situations, at least regarding porn, right? So what sort of assessment does someone need if they have questions or issues about porn? Here are some things I want to know during our first session:

1. Do they masturbate while watching porn? Do they enjoy it? Do they feel guilty about masturbating, as distinct from their feelings about porn?
2. If they're in, or have ever been in, a relationship, how do/did they function in it overall? If they've never been in a relationship, why not?
3. How do they function out in the world—at work or socially?
4. Do they feel or seem out of control in any other part of their lives?
5. What is their involvement in alcohol or drugs?
6. What prescription medications, if any, are they on?
7. Do they have a healthy relationship with the Internet in non-porn contexts?

You'll notice that only one of these questions is about pornography. That's because the basic aspects of people's problems involving pornography usually don't revolve around porn. So I want to know more about the *person*, which helps me understand the context, or meaning, of the porn-related behavior. This approach puzzles some guys, but they mostly feel relieved that I don't immediately jump on the omigod-it's-a-porn-problem bandwagon.

And yes, this comprehensive approach is in dramatic contrast to the porn addiction model, which starts, ends, and focuses on porn.

If it seems like a guy is mostly worrying in response to external pressure, treatment includes discussions about whether or not he is entitled to evaluate his porn-watching for himself, and whether there are other non-porn issues he needs to address (such as the power dynamics in his relationship, or his degree of assertiveness in life). Treatment often results in him reviewing his options for dealing with external pressure; clarification of his goals and values; and a sense that he's entitled to decide how he wants to live his life. He can then choose what he wants to do about his porn-watching.

If it seems like a guy is struggling more with internal pressure, our conversations focus on the dynamics of fear, anxiety, shame, and guilt, and how those might be mistaken for an actual problem. We talk about the nature of fantasy, and the importance of self-acceptance, especially around sexuality. Treatment often results in him reviewing his rigid, internal rules about things like masculinity, sexuality, fidelity, fantasy, or autonomy within a couple; again, he can then choose what he wants to do about his porn-watching.

Note that both groups of guys are more vulnerable to pressure (internal or external) because of America's PornPanic—which gives their decisions around porn, and others' judgements, an artificial sense of urgency. This, of course, makes it hard to think clearly. And PornPanic establishes other people and organizations as stakeholders in their personal porn habits. Suddenly, their porn-watching isn't private, but is something that others legitimately claim affects them.

When someone's problematic porn use interfaces with problems in other areas of their life—e.g., social isolation—it can easily look like they have a porn problem. Often, the more we discuss the life of someone with a so-called porn problem, the less likely it seems that their problem is porn. Unfortunately, PornPanic gets people so anxious and judgmental about porn that the non-porn issues of porn users get less attention than they should.

So as in many diagnostic evaluations, someone with an actual problem is often identified through a process of elimination. For example:

• Is the problem porn, or is it the Internet?

Many people get lost in the Internet; porn is the content for some, but if you take away porn, they'll stay lost in the Internet. The DSM-5 lists "Internet Gaming Disorder" as a condition needing further study. And there are now books, websites, and treatment programs for "Internet Addiction," considered by some to be a problem for millions of adults. I don't think "internet addiction" is a helpful model, but many people are way too attached to the internet.

Similarly, research reports[1] that half of American adults would "feel anxious" without their smartphone; although many people watch porn on them, even more people use them to check email compulsively. Most of us are prey to "variable ratio reinforcement"—we never know when we'll get a satisfying email, so we keep checking, over and over, regardless of consequences.

• Is the problem porn, or is it masturbation?

Of course, tens of millions of men and women masturbate weekly or daily without feeling any distress whatsoever. But some people masturbate only once a month and feel terribly guilty; others masturbate three or four times a day, and feel sore, confused, frustrated, or ashamed. These same people may not want sex with their mate, adding another layer of complexity to the situation.

• Is the problem porn, or is it the sexual dynamics in someone's life?

A porn user may be in a relationship that isn't sexually satisfying, whether in quantity, quality, or specific content. Or he may feel sexually inadequate, whether or not he has a classic sexual "dysfunction."

• Is the problem porn, or is porn being used to medicate anxiety, depression, loneliness, or anger?

This is far more common than the media, clinicians, or anti-porn activists realize. Whether accompanied by the reward of orgasm or not, watching porn can temporarily relieve uncomfortable internal states at virtually no immediate cost to the individual.

* * *

So what if a guy is concerned, and porn use isn't the real problem—it's just an expression of underlying issues? Then we'd expect the following:

a. Taking away the porn *won't solve the problem*. Indeed, that's what happens in porn addiction programs or "treatment" when you take the porn away. For example, men almost *never* have more sex with their wives or girlfriends simply because they stop watching porn.
b. Doing without the porn may be harder than anyone assumes (which may encourage the idea that porn is indeed the problem).
c. If people do give up porn they'll be disappointed when their deeper problem resurfaces, or new problems arise.
d. Getting the person to admit that there's something wrong with watching or being attached to porn probably won't help.
e. The person may have multiple problems that aren't even related to each other (e.g., depression and fear of his fantasies).

f. Whatever the actual problem is, it can be fixed without fixing the problematic porn use (which, ironically, may change in response to fixing
another problem).

g. The assessment may implicate other sexual expressions, such as strip clubs
or massage parlors.

h. A partner's self-righteous attitude may be implicated. Generally, this won't
be a helpful voice.

i. Some of the relationship's unspoken agreements may be implicated, such
as "We don't talk about sex" or "We pretend he's not bisexual."

j. There may be an inability to create meaningful emotional (or sexual) connection in the porn user, or his partner, or both.

Indeed, these possibilities are exactly what almost everyone (except those
stuck in the porn addiction model) has discovered about so-called porn issues.
"Porn issues" are, in fact, almost always secondary to other things, so treating them as a primary problem rarely works.

So if porn isn't the *real* problem when someone has issues with porn, what
are some of the likely issues?

From a psychological viewpoint, regularly masturbating to pornography
looks like a response to a wide range of situations, such as isolation, curiosity, anger, and guilt (as well as a simple desire for erotic pleasure). Whether
consciously or (more often) unconsciously, many emotional challenges end
up with men taking refuge in porn—whether or not they withdraw from their
partners emotionally or sexually. Let's look at some examples.

A. Everyone has emotional ups and downs. Some of us have more downs
than others, and some have more severe downs. Those downs can be varying
degrees of depression or anxiety, as well as related conditions like loneliness,
self-criticism, fear of the future, and feeling unattractive. We all need the ability to regulate our emotions; when we're strong enough, we do that through
positive self-talk ("tomorrow is another day"; "people still love me"; "that
was just bad luck").

At other times, we use less functional means to regulate our feelings, such
as snacking, drinking, flirting, shopping, or picking fights. The advantages
and disadvantages of each are fairly clear. For some people, masturbating to
porn is an important way to self-regulate. And like snacking or drinking, it
can be done in moderate ways or self-harming ways. When the only way that
people can medicate their feelings is by getting immersed in fantasy, that can
lead to trouble.

It's even more complicated when people struggle to keep their agreements
with themselves ("five more minutes and then I'll stop"). Of course, we're all
familiar with this experience—say, with cookies or Hulu episodes (one more

and then I'll go to bed). When the dysregulated activity is porn-watching, of course, there is far greater stigma.

B. What if someone's internal life is even more complicated? Some people struggle with what psychologist Doug Braun-Harvey calls internal erotic conflicts. Perhaps they feel ashamed of what gets them excited; at some point, even the shame itself may be part of the excitement. Psychologist Jack Morin called these "troublesome turn-ons." This may be true, for example, if a straight man fantasizes about sex with a man; or loves remembering secretly watching his grandmother getting undressed; or wants to explore a fetish or submission. For such a person, getting excited with porn may be the only way to manage their taboo eroticism.

For many of these guys, hiding their authentic eroticism from their partners seems crucial. They may see porn as enabling them to walk an erotic/shame tightrope: They get to have their excitement, while unconsciously criticizing it as "at least with porn I don't subject my beloved wife to my perverse preferences or fantasies."

C. Shame and fear of judgment are two key reasons that people unconsciously inhibit their arousal with a partner. And yet eroticism demands its day, so such a person may turn to porn for solo sex in which he can allow himself higher levels of excitement. Of course, if he lets himself get more excited with porn than with a partner, sex within the relationship can't possibly compete with masturbating to pornography.

There may be other reasons people don't become sufficiently excited with a partner. People are always blaming their partner for being insufficiently sexy or experimental, for not initiating, or for intruding on potential sexual moments with concerns about children or chores. Another reason is that people don't tell their partners what they like, or they don't find out what would motivate their partners sexually.

And of course some people are just wired with less capacity for arousal than others. Their chronic state of low arousal (and even anhedonia) may be temporarily "cured" by dramatic disinhibition—for which they give themselves permission when viewing porn. Because high arousal feels like being alive, there's an ongoing incentive to disinhibit—i.e., to view porn. In this sense, obsessive viewing can be seen as the result of the unending desire to feel alive.

I rarely see someone abandon a vibrant sex life for a private life of masturbation with porn.

However, when partner sex is boring or frustrating, porn can seem like an exciting alternative. The same can be true for someone who dislikes his partner's body. In fact, there are people for whom masturbating with porn is a desperate attempt to stay in a sexually unsatisfactory (or even sexless) marriage.

In this case it can be like an affair—the lesser of two evils, where ending the relationship would be more disruptive, painful, or damaging. And like affairs, by making the unbearable bearable, it can prolong an otherwise unacceptable situation.

D. A man's inadequate relationship with himself and his sexuality can make masturbating with porn seem like a safe alternative to the emotional risks of partner sex. A man may mistrust his sexuality, either because he's had too many scary experiences, or few or no experiences. He may fear that his sexuality will get out of control and overwhelm him, his partner, or both of them.

Some men don't know exactly who they are, sexually, so it's more emotionally comfortable to slide into an existing erotic structure (the world of porn) than to create their own. It's hard to be emotionally or sexually intimate when you don't have enough of a self.

Performance anxiety doesn't get mentioned often enough as a demotivator in a wide range of sexual and emotional situations. It's the main reason so many younger men use Viagra—"for insurance," they tell me. Even for men who have never had an actual problem, masturbation to porn is the only kind of sex in which they feel no performance (or other) anxiety. Some men who have had erection or ejaculation disappointments are, unfortunately, certain they can't satisfy a partner, so they settle into a lifestyle of solo sex.

Some therapists are keen to talk about "attachment" styles and inadequacy; they see porn use as an expression of poor attachment to a partner. While this isn't true for everyone who looks at porn, it is true for some—they just don't have the emotional skills or the adult desire to focus their sexual energies on one or more adults.[2]

On the other hand, columnist Dan Savage points out that many heterosexual men are angry at women, and that they enjoy porn where they can feel in control of a sexual situation, don't have to be attuned to a woman's needs or feelings, and can get pleasure watching videos of women being treated roughly. For men who are haunted by ambivalent feelings about women, who can't express reasonable resentment toward them, or who think of them as "other," watching porn can provide erotic experiences that help them avoid the complications of relating to a real person.

E. Has the guy had any sex-related trauma? Has he felt humiliated by an erection or ejaculation difficulty? Such events affect some men deeply. Because erection and ejaculation are involuntary, any experience suggesting they are unreliable or likely to go awry is a potential focus of anxiety.[3] It doesn't have to be this way; some men have one or two disappointing experiences with erection or ejaculation, then relax and move forward.

But given the typical definitions of sexual adequacy and masculinity for American men, many overgeneralize from a couple of (perhaps alcohol-fueled or simply circumstantial) erection "failures" and create anxiety—which, ironically, creates more of these "failures." From there it can be a short step to withdrawal from women and/or taking refuge in porn, in which anyone can feel confident. The viewer may symbolically absorb the obvious adequacy of the performers, much like consumers of adventure stories vicariously enjoy the hero's courage and strength.

Of course, some boys experience sexual exploitation or trauma, which can lead to sexual or intimacy problems in adulthood. Withdrawing into the controlled environment of masturbating to pornography can seem like the only safe erotic choice.

There's also the not-coercive-but-creepy erotic childhood experiences that are all too common—not just for girls, but for boys as well.

For example, there's lonely Mom continually confiding too much about her personal life to her son; there's intrusive Mom expressing way too much interest in son's toilet habits, genital development, masturbation, sexual fantasies, and adolescent exploits; there's licentious Dad encouraging son to be sexual before he's ready (and offering too much help in making it happen); there's neurotic Mom who's starting to feel old and unattractive, walking around the house half-undressed and wanting reassurance that she's still attractive; and there's narcissistic Dad who flaunts his sexual appeal, multiple affairs, or stream of inappropriate sexual commentary on every female who enters his field of vision, expecting his son to be a buddy and join in.

All of these can create unconscious reasons, later in life, to withdraw from sex with a partner, and/or prefer the safer, controlled, less-threatening idealizations of porn. Porn can be especially reassuring because the viewer can choose exactly what kinds of experiences he wants to have: No oversexed mothers for me! No performance pressure for me! No actual adult women with emotional needs, like my mother's that overwhelmed me when I was a child!

F. Finally, we should remember that there are guys out there who are clueless (their word, not mine) about women's bodies and sexuality. There are millions of adult virgins out there (not all of them engineers, although ironically a lot of men who develop the software and hardware that run the Internet are de facto virgins), and the Internet is perfectly designed for their primitive expressions of sexuality. Additionally, there are inexperienced men who scrutinize Internet porn to learn more about women and sex, to gain confidence and a program before their first partner encounter.

In a similar way, Internet porn can seem perfect for men with Asperger's Syndrome or ADHD. Their limited empathy or narrow emotional focus complicates both getting a partner and sharing sex, so masturbation to porn may be an ideal sexual environment. The repetition and predictability found in porn can be soothing, regardless of the content. For those with an incomplete sense of self, porn offers immersion in a ready-made world, almost like parking themselves on a conveyor belt, which carries them along without requiring too much of their own engagement.

And speaking of adaptation, we should mention the guy who spends hours with Internet porn—not watching, just collecting and sorting. Of course, when people spend time like this with stamps, baseball cards, Disney memorabilia, digital songs, or other non-sexual things, they're called hobbyists, which is generally considered a good thing—unless they lose touch with their loved ones, or job, school, or other responsibilities.

For some guys, collecting porn thumbnails is a symbolic way of trying to get the messy world of their sexuality under control, or perhaps a compulsive attempt to wrangle the Internet into a coherent, manageable suite. It often has little or nothing to do with orgasm or physical pleasure.

* * *

There's one more complication in deciding whether someone has a porn problem—the fact that a guy might prefer having a "porn problem" to another kind of problem, and therefore collude with his wife or others in his "diagnosis." For example, most people would rather do *anything* than tell their partner "I love you, but sex with you isn't much fun anymore," or "I feel so much pressure to make you orgasm from intercourse that it's hard to enjoy sex with you." Compared to those conversations, having a "porn problem" might seem quite acceptable.

SO WHAT IS A "PORN PROBLEM"? WHO HAS ONE?

Say a guy isn't compulsive with the Internet outside of porn; doesn't feel guilty about masturbating; isn't terrified of intimacy; feels good about himself and his sexuality. He doesn't like his porn habits, but he can't seem to change them. Should we say the guy has a porn problem?

Rather than "porn problem," I prefer the description "a problem expressed through porn use." It seems more accurate and more helpful in diagnosing or treating an actual problem.

America's PornPanic hates this textured and humanistic formulation, even though it's helpful in understanding and treating people's problems. PornPanic depends on the narrative that porn itself is a problem, exerting its destructive power by intruding into the lives of good people and their relationships. PornPanic demands a narrative that porn (that is, sex) undermines people's values and decision-making, rather than holding people responsible for their choices in a complicated world, part of whose complexity is our sexuality. This narrative helps demonize porn, helps diminish both male and female eroticism, and keeps moral entrepreneurs in business.

Many people have problems that they're expressing through their use of pornography. I'm sympathetic toward them (and their loved ones, if they're being affected), and I work hard every week to help them heal. To do that, it's important that I not get distracted by their porn use—and that I understand the bigger circumstances of their activity as best I can.

So how are problems expressed through porn use best treated? In this chapter we've looked at the many questions a skilled clinician would ask someone concerned about their porn use. When those questions reveal unresolved emotional issues (fear of intimacy, anxiety about perversion, belief that masturbation is harmful or offensive to God, etc.), the clinician can address them with his or her full inventory of clinical tools—assuming he or she is not distracted by the pornography aspect of a case.

That said, here are some goals I recommend for those struggling with unwanted or self-harming pornography use:

- Deciding it's OK to masturbate—with or without porn
- Finding other ways to regulate one's internal state, including medication
- Coming to terms with one's religious issues around sexuality
- Accepting one's sexual fantasies and preferences
- Resolving personal issues about sexual adequacy and "normalcy"
- Resolving internal erotic conflicts, reducing guilt and shame
- Diagnosing and treating any depressive, anxiety, mood, or attention disorders
- Repairing one's sex life with one's partner; this may involve recommitting to the relationship
- Talking honestly with one's partner about sex
- Learning to single-task during partner sex—i.e., to focus on nothing but the sex and your partner. The opposite of multi-tasking.

When issues such as these are resolved, an individual can decide exactly what relationship (if any) he would like to have with pornography, and what that looks like in his particular life.

Note that none of these includes the assessment that someone is bad, perverted, selfish, addicted, the wrong orientation, misogynist, sexually inadequate, potentially violent, or deserving punishment. The approaches discussed here are far more helpful and accurate.

Chapter Nine

WHY THERE'S NO SUCH THING AS PORN ADDICTION—AND WHY IT MATTERS

A "nymphomaniac" is a woman who has sex more than we think is OK.

A "porn addict" is a man who watches porn more than we think is OK.

Let's start with "addiction":

"I keep doing stupid things" is not an addiction.

"I swore to myself I wouldn't do it, but I did it" is not an addiction.

"Wow, the results of doing that were just as bad as everyone predicted" is not an addiction.

"I guess I didn't learn my lesson from doing it those other times" is not an addiction.

"I kept telling myself, 'don't do it, you'll regret it' and I did it anyway" is not an addiction.

"When I abstain from doing it, I feel deprived, crabby, and bored" is not an addiction.

Doing it, experiencing negative consequences, and doing it again is not an addiction.

If these things do, in fact, describe addiction, then the word "addiction" has lost its value. "Addiction" then just means repeating a bad choice, or making a stupid decision you later wish you hadn't, or making the same mistake over and over, or impulsively pursuing something now and regretting the consequences later.

If you call these experiences addiction, every person on earth is addicted to something. And yes, if these are your definitions of addiction, millions of Americans are afflicted with porn addiction.

But this is a particularly unhelpful definition of addiction, especially when it comes to pornography. Here are some problems with the disease of "porn addiction" (which was invented in the late 1990s as cybersex addiction):

- It pathologizes behavior that is often harmless—but which upsets someone other than the porn consumer himself.
- It is moralism pretending to be science. There is no consensus on what defines "porn addiction,"[1] nor on how to treat it, nor on what constitutes a successful cure—no porn? Some porn (how much?)? Only certain kinds of porn? Increased desire for one's partner?
- It overlooks/absolves the partners of porn users who might be contributing to a dysfunctional relationship in which high-volume porn use is an understandable response.
- It is contemptuous of masturbation; porn addicts are typically told they have to stop masturbating, or do it much less.[2]
- It prevents people with real, non-porn problems (like depression) from being identified and properly treated.
- If people do have a problem with porn, this approach keeps them from getting psychological and medical treatment that would actually be helpful.
- It honors "addicts" and their partners as the most knowledgeable people about the condition, reducing science to just another opinion. We don't do this with real diseases like diabetes or heart disease.
- It ignores the extent to which someone's porn problem might actually be an unhealthy attachment to Internet use.
- There are no withdrawal symptoms when someone discontinues using porn. They might be crabby (especially if they've given up masturbation), but their body doesn't shake, sweat, or get clammy, they don't suffer muscle aches, loss of appetite, nausea, or vomiting, and they don't experience nightmares, paranoia, or crying spells. That's what withdrawal is like from any real addiction.
- People who claim to treat "porn addiction" rarely offer a model of healthy porn use.
- If porn consumers/addicts really needed to increase their dose over time (the classical definition of addiction), they'd all quit their school/jobs and spend all their time masturbating to porn, which is clearly not true.

So how did we get here? Historically speaking, America got to porn addiction via sex addiction.

Sex addiction was invented in the 1980s by addictionologist (*not* sex therapist, thank you) Patrick Carnes.[3] Lacking professional training in sexuality, he mistakenly said that people who feel out of control around sex *are* out of control around sex. He defined that as addiction, and off we went.

Carnes was very familiar with America's existing infrastructure for treating alcoholics: AA groups, the 12 steps, sponsorship structure, programs for spouses, and in-patient treatments, all ready to welcome new addicts. People ashamed and self-critical about their sexuality loved the welcoming narcissistic nourishment ("we've been waiting for YOU!") that came with admitting their sex addiction. They were told exactly what to do, cheered when they did it, and forgiven when they didn't. The sex addiction movement replaced their perceived moral degeneracy, impulsivity, selfishness, and self-indulgence with the dignity of a disease, fellowship with millions of other addicts (alcoholic and otherwise), and sympathy for their plight.

This movement offered little real understanding of sexuality—if anything, its message was that addicts needed to focus on sex much less, making sexual feelings, desires, and experiences a smaller part of their lives. Even today, 30 years later, people who "treat" sex addiction are rarely sex therapists, and they discourage sexual expression that is lusty, complex, or non-traditional.

For alcoholics and drug addicts who were old-timers in AA, sex addiction was a chance to work the steps again. Even if an alcoholic didn't feel out of control sexually, feeling uncomfortable or regretful about sex was enough to qualify for participation. Just as with alcohol, so as with sex—if you want membership in the fellowship of addicts, come on in—no screening necessary.

And a series of celebrities caught doing things they regretted were deciding that they were sex addicts—such as Michael Douglas, Mike Tyson, Marion Barry, and Rob Lowe. So sex addiction was just sitting there—endorsed by Oprah, although rarely by actual sex therapists—when broadband porn hit the country in 2000. Predictably, some people would misuse porn, or feel confused by it, or upset their partner with it. And these were potential customers for the emotional safety net provided by the porn addiction movement. Why be an isolated selfish bastard or confused person or frustrated spouse when you could have a disease with a welcoming fellowship?

And so today, millions of people are said to suffer with porn addiction.[4] And although most sex therapists don't use the concept and therefore say they've never seen a case of it, that hasn't stopped various religious, clinical, online, and criminal justice institutions from quickly developing treatment programs, including incredibly lucrative in-patient programs.

DSM-5

The porn addiction gravy train has been slowed down a bit by once again losing the struggle for inclusion in the updated DSM-5, in 2013. How was the decision to exclude it made? Or put another way, why did the most prestigious body of psychiatrists in the world decide that neither "sex addiction" nor "porn addiction" were fit to include in the worldwide manual of mental disorders?

The review process to update the DSM-IV took more than a decade and involved thousands of professionals.[5] After sifting through mountains of data, opinions, and clinical charts, the review panel of experts decided that "there is insufficient peer-reviewed evidence to establish the diagnostic criteria and course descriptions needed" to include sex addiction or porn addiction as actual disorders.[6]

Refusing to recognize and include porn addiction in the DSM is no small thing—the DSM includes everything from A to Z (well, A to V), from ADHD to Voyeurism, from Acute Stress Disorder to Vascular Neurocognitive Disorder.

The review committee noted that there is no recognized consensus on criteria for the alleged disease of porn addiction, its symptoms, typical trajectory, effective treatments, etc. Reflecting this, a recent review published in *Current Sexual Health Reports* says that only 27 percent of all *peer-reviewed* articles on porn addiction contained any actual data (which tells you about the low level of science in the new sex addiction "journals.")[7]

Similarly, there has never been a protocol for differential diagnosis for porn addiction. How exactly should a clinician distinguish Porn Addiction from, say, Depressive Disorder; Anxiety Disorder; Obsessive-Compulsive Disorder; Bipolar Disorder; or Post-Traumatic Stress Disorder? Because the symptoms of porn addiction often look like the symptoms of these various well-established and well-studied mental disorders, DSM investigators were required to find important ways to differentiate porn addiction from them. They couldn't, which discouraged committee members from including it as a new diagnosis.

There was also the issue that a lot of porn addiction is self-diagnosed or partner-diagnosed.[8] This would never be considered appropriate for, say, bipolar disorder (much less for diabetes). Tellingly (though not surprisingly), those self-diagnosing as porn addicts are disproportionately men whose religious values conflict with their self-reported sexual behavior and desires.[9]

SO WHAT IS REAL ADDICTION?

When your body has changed its way of metabolizing a substance such that your decision-making is compromised, *that's* addiction. Think alcohol. Heroin. Pain-killers like OxyContin.

Nicotine is another example of real addiction: In the United States, less than 7 percent of people are able to quit smoking on any given attempt without medicines or other help. Even with medicine, only 25 percent of smokers can stay smoke-free for over six months. And that's only six months.[10] Similarly, the British Heart Foundation (BHF) found that 82 percent of smokers have unsuccessfully tried to quit at least once. Dr. Mike Knapton, Associate Medical Director for the BHF, says: "Every year more than 100,000 [British] smokers die because of their addiction."[11]

Unlike pornography, substances like crack cocaine and tobacco are actually addictive. No one leaves a great sex life for porn. But some people *do* leave a great life for heroin, alcohol, and truly addictive substances *because they're addicted.*

The simplistic argument that porn is like drugs and therefore works like drugs is just silly. An analogy is not evidence. Flour looks like cocaine, but they work differently. Jogging and talking to the police both make you sweat, but the activities are very different, and your body even experiences them differently.

After taking up addictive substances like crack cocaine, users soon stop experiencing any pleasure from using—only normalcy when using, and relief from the distress of not using. Masturbating to porn is different from addictive substances in that it continues to be enjoyable over many years; anyone who doesn't get pleasure from using porn almost always stops looking at it. If they don't, that's a sign of a recognizable and treatable psychological problem, such as OCD or PTSD.

DOES USING PORN LEAD TO ERECTILE DYSFUNCTION?

The newest entry in the porn-is-a-dangerous-product sweepstakes is the mythical disease of PIED—Porn Induced Erectile Dysfunction. Using a combination of misleading junk neuroscience, testimonials, and the old news that virtually all men occasionally don't get erections when they want them, anti-porn forces have concluded that masturbating to high-speed porn (there's that pesky masturbation behavior again), especially if you start young, actually affects your ability to get erect with a live partner.

These alarmist activists conveniently overlook factors such as:

- Young people have unrealistic expectations about the conditions under which they're likely to get (or not get) erect
- The medical definition of Erectile Dysfunction (ED), which requires a lack of alcohol, lack of performance anxiety, and recurring symptoms, not just the occasional disappointment

- Today's decreasing level of live preparation for partner sexual interactions that young people get (leading to unrealistic expectations, having sex under sub-optimal conditions, and insufficient tools to deal with the results)
- The way 24-hour Internet connectivity can make every part of real life seem routine and boring

Nevertheless, even television personality Dr. Oz (again, no training in sexuality) is concerned about supposed PIED. He bases his concern on three main things:

1. A one-time Italian study that wasn't peer-reviewed and has never been replicated.
2. Testimonials of young (they're always young) men who claim that they had ED, that porn caused it, and that abstaining from porn fixed it.
3. The fact that his TV audience is almost entirely female, and that any show with the word "erection" in it gets a ratings spike. In fact, he did four shows on this in February 2013—"sweeps month" in industry jargon, when ratings are measured for advertisers.[12]

The experts on these Dr. Oz episodes disagreed with each other, and with the newly minted orthodoxy of the PIED movement. Urologist Dr. Andrew Kramer said that men with PIED need four pornless weeks to "reboot," while the PIED movement says six months or even a year is usually needed. On the other hand, sexologist Ian Kerner said that PIED might come from sexual boredom (in which case it wouldn't be PIED), and that treating PIED is "not about cutting out the porn," but perhaps using a different kind of porn. So PIED is a supposed problem whose believers can't even agree on its contours, much less the contours of healthy sexuality.

Where is the actual data showing an increase in young men's erectile problems? It doesn't exist. Although popular jokes suggest that only middle-aged and older men have erection problems, scientists have known for at least 60 years that at least 10 percent of men age 29 and younger have erectile dissatisfaction.[13] While there was no Internet for young people to share their erection woes back then, that reality has been mentioned for dozens of centuries by writers including Shakespeare, Chaucer, and Aristophanes. People unfamiliar with world history or world literature think that erection problems, and sexual problems in general, are primarily a modern phenomenon (just like many young people in the 1960s thought they invented sexual ecstasy).

I started practicing sex therapy 20 years before Internet porn became ubiquitous, and I haven't seen any increase in erection problems in the 15 years since Internet porn came into every home. Neither have any of the urologists, psychologists, or sex therapists with whom I work.

To support this professional experience, science offers studies thousands of miles apart. For example, North American neuroscientists Prause and Pfaus recently wrote of their research, in which pornography use was related to greater sexual desire for one's partner, not to ED or lower desire.[14] An ocean away, European researchers Landripet and Stulhofer found that neither frequency of porn viewing nor changes in the frequency of use were related to erectile problems.[15] Both studies were published in a prestigious medical journal. Together, these two studies refute claims that watching porn desensitizes erectile function, which supposedly leads to decreased desire and arousal for partner sex.

It is true that more young men are using erection drugs now than when they first came out.[16] Blame a culture obsessed with intercourse, in which everyone wants the best erection they can get. Blame women who, more empowered than two decades ago, are voicing dissatisfaction in sexual situations where they didn't used to complain. Blame porn that shows every man always erect (and, Mr. Porn Consumer, how do you suppose that happens?). Blame a young adult culture that sees Viagra as part of the "insurance" package they want before starting sexual encounters in which they feel anxious—and blame young men's learned ability to fake the symptoms of ED in order to get Viagra.[17]

If there is an increase in erection problems among Millennials, one likely explanation is that today's drug of choice for young singles is alcohol, which undermines erections far more than marijuana did when it was young people's favorite drug in the '60s. People who have had a lot to drink are more likely to feel anxious (and therefore more likely to have erection problems) than people who have smoked a lot of marijuana.

Possibly the most important issue here is the extent to which young people live on Internet-enabled devices: occupied with literally hundreds of texts per day, rapidly switching between screens, swiping between images, looking for facts or answers before trying to remember them, imagine them, or discuss them with a live companion. It isn't that sex can't compete with porn—**sex can't compete with the Internet. Sex can't be as compelling, as varied, as unpredictable, as moment-to-moment rewarding as the Internet.** Contrasted with this daily opulent online experience, young people tell me there simply isn't enough going on during actual sex to absorb their attention. *That's* what limits arousal and erection far more than the content of what they look at, whether it's porn or anything else.

All of which is different than saying there's a neurological pathway through which porn use undermines erections.

And do remember that there is no reliable data showing an increase in erection problems today over yesterday.

Most men who swear off porn also cut out (or reduce) masturbation. Whatever improvements they notice in their erections are undoubtedly more because of not masturbating (or increased talking with their partners, or recommitting to sex in their relationship) than because of not watching porn. For many men, reduction of masturbation will increase sex drive, which over time can result in more morning erections and even nocturnal emissions. Most men would say that giving up masturbation is a pretty high price to pay for wet pajamas.

Let's remember that young people are not experts in sexuality, not even experts in young people's sexuality. We do know that most 23-year-olds are trying to grow up and understand sexuality. Most do a poor job of it, and when older, disown much of their own 23-year-old's behavior and beliefs. Choosing masturbation with porn instead of risking sex with a live woman is only the latest version of this. Ask a bunch of today's 40-year-olds how they feel about their sexual decisions and beliefs back when they were 23—and most will roll their eyes and shudder, laugh, or both. If you're 40, or when you become 40, this will presumably be true for you, too.

WHAT ABOUT NEUROSCIENCE?

"Non-experts really love explanations from neuroscience, even if they're wrong," says psychologist Carol Tavris. The fast-evolving technology in brain-imaging techniques has practically hypnotized laypeople—especially journalists—with images that are both stunning and incomprehensible. Still, Tavris says, "Many people regard evidence from brain images as being more 'real' than other types of psychological information."[18]

Other scientists have noted this effect as well. Three recent experiments tested the hypothesis that brain images have a particularly persuasive influence on the public perception of research on cognition. The results: "[P]resenting brain images with articles summarizing cognitive neuroscience research resulted in higher ratings of scientific reasoning for arguments made in those articles, as compared to articles accompanied by bar graphs, a topographical map of brain activation, or no image.

"We argue that brain images are influential because they provide a physical basis for abstract cognitive processes, appealing to people's affinity for reductionistic explanations of cognitive phenomena." Or as Tavris puts it, brain images satisfy the public's preference for "neat" biological explanations over "messy" psychological rationale."[19]

Having said that, what do those imaging studies say about the brains of people who watch porn? Do they look like the brains of people on crack cocaine? If so, doesn't that prove that porn is destructive and even addictive?

"Watching the NCAA playoffs is going to change your brain, eating chocolate—any time you have any kind of experience, it's going to change your brain," says Rory C. Reid, a research psychologist at UCLA's Neuropsychiatric Institute who is also an expert in hypersexual behavior. He's hardly pro-porn—"Philosophically, I've got all sorts of problems with porn"—but as a scientist, he says, "[T]his idea that consumption of pornography causes cortical atrophy that leads to negative consequences? We haven't seen that."[20]

Similarly, Bruce Carpenter, a researcher at Brigham Young University—yes, *that* Brigham Young—is morally opposed to pornography. He suspects that "pornography has larger deleterious effects upon individuals, family, and society," but adds: "Now to the evidence. THERE IS NONE . . . There is not a single study of pornography use showing brain damage or even brain changes."[21]

Dr. Barry Komisaruk, a Rutgers University psychologist who has done groundbreaking neuroscience research on the brain during orgasm, also says that there are no studies demonstrating that porn's effect on the brain is anything resembling addiction.[22]

And yet periodically one reads a headline and lead like the following, from 2013:

"Pornography addiction leads to same brain activity as alcoholism or drug abuse, study shows." *Cambridge University scientists reveal changes in brain for compulsive porn users which don't occur in those with no such habit.*[23]

Cambridge—that's like the gold standard of universities, right? So doesn't this seal the deal on the reality of porn addiction?

Not at all—once we look at the actual science. According to neuroscientist James Pfaus, Professor at the Center for Studies in Behavioral Neurobiology at Montreal's Concordia University, "Assuming that it eventually passes peer review, all this study shows is that the nucleus accumbens (ventral striatum) is activated by *preferred* visual erotica. This happens with most preferred stimuli, including pictures of one's favorite foods, preferred music, photos of your newborn baby, etc. And yes, it also happens in drug addicts with photos of preferred drugs or drug paraphernalia. You would not regard the chills I get listening to the final chorale from Bach's 'St. Matthew's Passion' (and that lights up my ventral striatum like Vegas) as an indication that I am suffering from 'music addiction.' "

Continues Pfaus, "Correlation is *not* evidence of causality, no matter what a newspaper headline says. The notion that so-called 'porn addiction' *leads* to brain activity is not at all what these data show. They show only that watching preferred visual erotica activates that region, whereas watching non-preferred visual erotica (in the matched controls) activates it less. Again, this is the case when *many* biologically relevant stimuli are preferred."[24]

To pick just one of many such examples, a recent study[25] shows that even the smell of newborn babies triggers the same reward centers as drugs. That is, when women catch the scent of a newborn baby, their dopamine pathways in a region of the brain associated with reward learning light up. The same dopamine surge is also associated with satiating sexual and drug-addiction cravings. This mechanism influences us by triggering "the motivation to act in a certain way because of the pleasure associated with a given behavior."

What makes some substances addictive is that they always shift brain response to craving states rather than liking states. As neurobiologists Georgiadis and Kringelbach point out, "In no case has a shift away from liking to wanting or craving been demonstrated" with pornography . . . [N]o data have demonstrated that [porn] is different from any other 'liked' activity or object."[26]

After reviewing the literature of the neuroimaging studies of the human sexual response cycle, Georgiadis and Kringelbach further "normalized" sexual arousal with pornography, concluding "it is clear that the networks involved in human sexual behavior are remarkably similar to the networks involved in processing other rewards."[27]

To be fair, while the media and anti-porn activists are creating impressive headlines out of preliminary studies with low numbers and few if any controls, the scientists doing the studies rarely make the massive claims that non-experts do. Neuroscientists themselves generally say they don't know what brain activation maps mean in terms of subjective experience, certainly not about decision-making. Beware non-neuroscientists' claims about what neuroscience means.

If the junk neuroscience of anti-porn activists was accurate, some 30–40 million American porn users would end up crippled (they obviously don't), simultaneously losing interest in sex and wanting more intense sexual experiences (I know, it makes no sense). And all porn users, needing a bigger and bigger dose of their porn "drug," would end up pursuing the ultimate in novel porn experiences—bestiality and kiddie porn. Of course, the overwhelmingly common outcome is that that doesn't happen.

Marnia Robinson (an attorney) and her husband Gary Wilson (a self-described neuroscience enthusiast) have made their name promoting the idea that neuroscience proves that masturbation to pornography actually induces erectile dysfunction, loss of desire for partner, and addiction. Until it was terminated in 2014, their *Psychology Today* blog continually argued that the brains of addicted men become desensitized to sexual stimulation and so they must continually seek novelty via porn that is more extreme, involves fetishes, or is even the "wrong" orientation. Other movements promoting this idea include No-Fap, YourBrainOnPorn, RebootNation, and XXXChurch. Interestingly, all these people are non-psychologists, non-therapists, and non-sexologists. These various websites and movements expose their ignorance of sexuality by saying things such as:

- Orgasm is the reward from watching porn [*not always*], and the greater the number of hours watched, the more orgasms a person has [*not true*]; and orgasm is "the most powerful natural dopaminergic reward in the nervous system."[28] [*really not true*]
- People should only watch porn that strictly reflects their own sexual orientation [*1. Why? 2. This ignores the fact that most heterosexual men and women periodically enjoy same-gender fantasies*]. Otherwise they're vulnerable to a supposedly new syndrome, homosexual obsessive compulsive disorder (HOCD).
- People who have a single extramarital affair and thereby risk their marriage are sex addicts.[29] [*1. What? 2. Presumably, Dr. Hall feels the same way about people who watch porn despite inviting conflict and risk into their marriages.*]

Just in case you are not a neuroscientist, let me help you make sense of all this new brain research, junk and otherwise:

- The studies are on tiny populations.
- The studies *can't* show causality, only correlation (legitimate scientists always say this; journalists and porn addictionologists rarely do).
- Studies don't look at possible distinctions between people who look at a lot of porn *without problems* and people who look at a lot of porn either compulsively or with problematic outcomes.
- The argument is circular. Of *course* people who use a lot of porn are more excited when they look at porn, compared with people who don't use a lot of porn. You could do the same study with people who do and don't like vanilla milkshakes and get the identical result.
- There's no explanation of people who watch a medium or large amount of porn for years without becoming addicted, compulsive, self-destructive, or sexually dysfunctional.
- The argument is "heads I win, tails you lose": if the brain activation in the high-porn (very small) group is higher, it supposedly shows addiction. If the brain activity in the high-porn use group is lower, it's described as "reduced sensitivity" or "hypo-reactivity" in the brains of compulsive porn users.

On the other hand, if a classical addiction model is really at work here, we would expect compulsive porn users to show *less* brain activation over time rather than more, due to increased tolerance of the addictive substance (porn).

The field of brain research relevant to this matter is in its infancy. Science still has little idea about exactly what and how the brain does what it does. So virtually any neuroscientific outcome can be interpreted as supporting some ideology or other.

Non-scientists Robinson and Wilson keep forgetting two basic scientific principles:

- Correlation doesn't equal causation.
- The plural of "anecdote" is not "data."

CAN YOU PROVE THERE'S NO SUCH THING AS PORN ADDICTION?

No. But that's not my job (or yours). It's the job of people who believe that porn addiction exists to prove that there is such a thing. They can't. What they can do is show how some kinds of porn use are *like* addictive activities. But reasoning like that doesn't prove anything. For now, we have perfectly adequate models to explain various kinds of repetitive, compulsive, ritualistic, or self-destructive porn use, such as:

- Psychological problems like obsessive-compulsive disorder, bipolar disorder, depression, or Asperger's Syndrome
- Guilt or shame that keeps driving someone back to images they find troubling
- Strong sexual curiosity that has no other outlet, often combined with secrecy or isolation
- Inhibited sexual communication of either an individual or a couple
- Dissatisfaction with the sex life available to someone, whether they are single or coupled
- PTSD or other intense reasons for turning away from intimate relationships or partner sex

And let's remember that millions and millions of people look at a lot of porn every single week and don't think they have a problem.

Do some consumers have a problem with porn? Of course. But "problematic" is not the same as "addictive;" because they're treated quite differently, we shouldn't mistake the first for the second. And if the porn addiction movement is using "porn addiction" metaphorically, they should either put the phrase in quotes or stop using it.

"PORN ADDICTION" IS PART OF TODAY'S PORNPANIC

As part of transforming pornography from immoral habit to dangerous substance, activists have had to relentlessly describe porn as spectacularly unsafe. Calling it addictive was brilliant—it facilitates insidious comparisons with drugs that everyone agrees are toxic, such as heroin. And by calling it addictive, AA and other existing treatment agencies could be mobilized to help those concerned about it—and to offer alleged expertise regarding sexual phenomena about which they know nothing.

Here's how one advocate of the porn addiction model describes the allegedly inevitable outcomes now challenging America:

> *Normal men become addicted to porn,*
> *Which leads to sexual dysfunction,*
> *Which leads to losing interest in real women.*
> *Through porn addiction, men craving a fix (porn) also learn to see women as nothing more than objects for their pleasure.*
> *They dehumanize women, thus becoming desensitized to their pain at being trafficked. "Thus, porn creates the demand for sex trafficking."*[30]

This bizarre chain of illogic is a textbook expression of the porn addiction model. It fits perfectly with the myth that all porn is violent, and with the woman-hating, man-hating, and sex-hating belief that watching porn is a form of violence against women.

As discussed elsewhere, the "addiction" model allowed for self-diagnosis and self-referral; thus, guilt, shame, and anxiety were valuable in helping people recruit themselves. Addiction recovery groups offer themselves as a place for people to lose their guilt and shame; sexual shame being as toxic as it is, confessing to an "addiction" must seem like a trivial price to pay for relief from painful emotions, regardless of whether behavior changes or not.

The addiction model also values testimonials as evidence—which, in fact, is the only "evidence" available to the anti-porn movement. Science? Who needs science? Stories of recovering men and harmed women are presented as sufficient evidence that porn is a magic poison constituting a significant threat to people and communities. Counter-testimonials, of course, are ignored. No one who believes in porn addiction can account for the 30 or 40 million regular porn users whom no one says are addicts.

As befits a PornPanic, the new concept of porn as toxic substance contains no model of healthy porn use. Porn addicts are encouraged to get and stay "sober" forever—hardly the "teach a man to fish" routine we hear so much about.

There's also tremendous confusion about whether porn addicts should be allowed to masturbate without porn. No one has yet coherently explained why a porn addict can't masturbate to just his own fantasies—the PornPanic has rendered even something that isn't porn (and indeed, predates it both developmentally and technologically) unclean and dangerous. If a porn addict *can* masturbate to just his own imagination, how is that different from masturbating to porn?

For that matter, many porn addiction programs aren't too keen on masturbating anyway; for example, NoFap hosts challenges "in which participants abstain from porn and masturbation to recover from porn addiction and compulsive sexuality."[31]

The porn addiction movement seems unfamiliar with the typical ecology of porn-watching and sexual relationships. Here are "symptoms" of porn addiction, followed by non-addiction explanations involving rather ordinary sexuality:

Symptom: "Escalation" of use
Explanation: I like it, and want more.

Symptom: Loss of attraction to partner
Explanation: A very common occurrence in long-term relationships regardless of porn use or non-use.

Symptom: In a 2012 study, about 20 percent of participants said that they preferred the excitement of watching porn to being sexually intimate with their partner.[32]
Explanation: At least 20 percent of all coupled people would rather do *anything* than have sex with their partner—because sex with their partner isn't that compelling, they're chronically upset with their partner, or they're uncomfortable getting that close to their partner. Whether such a person would rather garden or watch porn is irrelevant.

Symptom: Crabbiness when one attempts to quit porn (and therefore quit masturbation)
Explanation: Most people are crabby if they relinquish a substantial part (or all) of their sex life.

Symptom: Content of porn changes over time
Explanation: The healthy human brain craves novelty. That's why we buy new stuff when we don't need it, go to new restaurants, want to listen to new music when we already love our old favorites, and yearn to travel to unfamiliar places. We want different porn just like we want different sex; for those in monogamous relationships, experiencing different porn is far easier than creating different partnered sex (whether within the couple or outside it).

Symptom: Using porn despite negative consequences
Explanation: Human life commonly involves people making decisions whose consequences they don't like.

WHY DOES IT MATTER WHAT WE CALL IT?

Words are how we both describe and understand reality. Most people agree—now—that there's a difference between calling a woman "frigid" and saying a woman is picky about with whom she has sex. In 100 years, people will look back on today's concepts and words like "porn addiction" the way we now look back on previously legitimate words and ideas like "witch," "possessed by the devil," "a woman's place," "henpecked," and "past-life regression."

Of course it matters what we call things. If words didn't matter, we wouldn't now be using expressions like "the N word" or "F-bomb." And we would still be saying "drunken bum" instead of "alcoholic."

Chapter Ten

INCREASING PORN LITERACY AND SEXUAL INTELLIGENCE FOR THERAPISTS, DOCTORS, AND CLERGY

Let's be honest: Like every profession, counseling has a range of practitioners—some adequate, some excellent, some mediocre. More than almost any other profession, however, who the counselor *is* determines the kind of professional he or she is going to be.

Nowhere is that more true than when the topic is sexuality. In fact, when the topic is pornography, there are some counselors whose sessions are worse than no counseling at all. There, I've said it. As we're always telling our clients, acknowledging a problem is the first step toward solving it.

Let me introduce you to four professionals who do more damage than good as they handle cases involving pornography:

• David, a psychologist in Colorado

After months and months of quarrelling, they finally go to a marriage counselor—which just about destroys their marriage.

The wife leads. "We're here to find out if his porn-watching is a form of infidelity."

That isn't why I'm here, the husband thinks.

"It's completely disrupted our sex life."

No it hasn't, he thinks. You have.

"So," asks the psychologist, "If your porn-watching is tearing the marriage apart, why won't you stop?"

- **Tyrone, a pastoral counselor in Rhode Island**

"When you watch all that porn, I wonder if you love me anymore," the girl-friend says sadly. "Why else would you leave me like that?"

The therapist jumps right in and faces the boyfriend. "You'll have to choose what you love more—your porn or your girlfriend."

This is a ridiculous choice, he thinks. Of course he loves his girlfriend more. He loves her more than he loves coffee, too, but he doesn't think he needs to give up coffee to prove it.

- **Monika, a sex therapist in California**

Ultimately, marriage counselor and wife agree: his porn use has no legitimacy. No wonder he feels they're ganging up on him. And no wonder the couple becomes increasingly alienated from each other. The therapist has taken a pair of marital allies with a disagreement and turned them into adversaries. Suddenly he's fighting for the right to be himself, to be an adult—a much more serious challenge than any mere disagreement about porn.

- **Cherisse, a social worker in Michigan**

The therapist puts it simply: "You're a porn addict. You won't even stop watching when it's killing the wife you say you love."

Killing her? What about the other 99 percent of their life together? When they're not arguing about porn it's pretty nice—at least it was until they started therapy.

"This is fundamental," the therapist challenges the wife. "If you want this infidelity to stop, demand it. Tell him you forbid this disgusting insult in your house." And so she does.

What he hears is: I don't count. My needs are not as important as my wife's. So I must keep my activity a secret.

This erodes any desire he has left for her. And so this pathetic excuse for marriage counseling drives the couple further apart.

Pornography use has become one of the central counseling issues of our time. Unfortunately, our culture does not support counseling professionals in doing their most effective work in this area. And as America's PornPanic gets more emotional and more politicized every day, damaging sessions like those excerpted here are becoming increasingly common. The siren call of the well-funded and publicly accepted porn addiction movement makes our job even more difficult.

If you want to be helpful with these cases, you have to find out why, exactly, clients have come to see you. "Too much porn" (like "too much spending" or "always criticizing") is too vague to be a true clinical project. "I feel guilty about what I watch" or "I feel too angry about his porn to have sex with him" are clinical dilemmas worth addressing. And although porn may be the center of where you start a case, it should rarely be where you end up with it.

American culture is ambivalent about pornography: almost all men interested in sex consume it, yet most hide this, deny it, and feel shame about it. Women who think about their mate using porn often feel powerless, confused, or resentful. Other women ignore the whole cultural phenomenon and assume their mate doesn't watch porn. Many parents of teen boys or girls make the same mistaken assumption: "Porn? Be serious—not *my* kid."

This cultural ambivalence creates a special complication for clinicians: What end-states are we aiming toward? How much of the problem is people's behavior, and how much is their *feelings* about their behavior (or each other's behavior)? To make things more complex, when it comes to the Internet, what counts as "behavior" anyway?

We now live in a digital world, which didn't exist in its present form when you were being trained. *Of course* people are using digital media for sexual purposes. The niche possibilities of Internet pornography (as opposed to mass-produced magazine porn) have revealed a stunning breadth of fetishes and fantasies that most people had no clue existed. Neither clinical nor pastoral training prepare young professionals for the foot fetishes, crushies, furries, chubby chasers, waist trainers, leather daddies, frotteurists, transsexuals, or bears and cubs that are now routine on porn websites.

Naturally, ordinary people are bringing their incomplete personal and couples' skills to this new digital playground, creating the same old human problems, albeit with more colorful details.

Those problems are our area of expertise. So you don't need to be an expert in every exotic kind of porn in order to do good work around this topic. Just treat these clients as you treat all others: with dignity, a non-judgmental attitude, an openness to learning, and a desire to know what meaning and value clients give to their experiences and feelings.

What are people talking about when they're talking about pornography? Here are some topics you can expect to discuss in these cases:

- Wanting to increase one's sexual desire
- Wanting to increase one's partner's desire
- Mourning one's partner's lack of interest
- Wanting to enjoy the state of arousal
- Wanting to enjoy a more intense state of arousal
- Wanting to validate one's ability to get aroused
- Arousal as an antidote to boredom, low self-esteem, hopelessness, or anger
- Porn-watching as habitual
- Porn-watching as a high-integrity way of staying in a sexless marriage

- Porn-watching as an alternative to going to a sex worker
- Porn-watching as a battleground for internal conflict
- Porn-watching as a solution to spiritual restlessness
- Porn-watching as medication for depression, anxiety, or isolation

When pornography is part of individual or couples counseling it can be so distracting that we forget some basic principles of counseling. Here they are, applied to cases involving porn.

• Don't take sides.

The cardinal rule of couples counseling is to not take sides. Some counselors have trouble following this high standard when the subject is sex, all the more so when a case involves pornography. Remember that the pain of the porn consumer's partner is no more important than the dignity and needs of the porn consumer. As you know, when one partner is more upset or vocal than the other, we must be vigilant not to side with him/her, regardless of the topic.

• Remember to do a differential diagnosis.

Some people who use pornography in a self-defeating way have serious emotional issues. These can include bipolar disorder, depression, obsessive-compulsive disorder, anxiety, PTSD, borderline personality, autism/Asperger's, antisocial personality, or intermittent explosivity.

Other problems may involve alcohol or substance abuse, chronic physical pain, low self-esteem, or undiagnosed effects of prescription medication. And some may be crushed by the feeling that God hates or has abandoned them.

Make sure you assess for emotional, environmental, medical, and historical issues before you treat a problem presented as involving pornography.

• Don't depend on common cultural myths about porn.

For a list of common myths, and facts on which you can rely, see Chapter 3.

• Do know your values around masturbation, infidelity, and lust.

Everyone is entitled to their own values. If yours don't leave you the option of being patient, empathic, and non-judgmental about issues relating to a client's porn use, both you and the client will be better served by you referring the case on to a colleague.

• Don't get involved with what's "normal."

For years, every one of our clients has been hearing what's sexually normal—from Oprah, from their parents, from *Cosmo* or *Men's Health*, from their faith tradition, from their friends or brother-in-law, and yes, indirectly from porn. They don't need one more voice in this chorus.

Besides, the goal of all counseling is to empower clients to know their values and to act on them with integrity. That's "their values," not what's "normal." That's "integrity," not what's "normal."

When it comes to sexuality, there is no normal; when it comes to sexual fantasy, to be outside what others consider normal might be part of the fantasy. Whether your goal is to support or to influence clients, getting rid of the concept of sexually "normal" is crucial.

• Don't be in love with porn addiction (or sex addiction).

There is no evidence that "porn addiction" exists; indeed, both it and sex addiction were rejected from both the DSM-5 and ICD-10 (the international medical classification published by WHO, the World Health Organization). A key problem with the porn addiction model is its assumption that porn consumers have lost control of their decision-making, which is rarely true; when it is true, it's almost always part of a syndrome that's far larger than porn, such as bipolar disorder or major depression.

Making repetitive decisions despite negative consequences does not mean that someone is out of control or addicted. And do keep in mind that *feeling* out of control is not the same as *being* out of control. For more on the important subject of "porn addiction," see page 159.

• Don't assume you know what porn use means to this person at this time.

Disrespect for his wife? Expression of insecurity? Commitment to stay in a sexless marriage? Wrestling with shame about taboo fantasies? Something else entirely? We have no idea until we ask, listen, and ask some more.

Any source that states "porn use *always* means such-and-such" should be disregarded for that statement alone.

• Remember that fantasy generally doesn't predict behavior.

We all know that in non-sexual arenas, fantasy rarely predicts behavior. People commonly fantasize about robbing a bank, killing their boss, giving their children to Mark Zuckerberg—and yet they rarely do so. It's the same with porn. Porn reflects fantasy far, far more than it reflects desire. And it predicts behavior even less. Just as porn isn't a documentary, don't assume that a given client's porn preferences are a literal depiction of their sexual preferences, or how they wish to relate to women, men, or sex.

A substantial number of women enjoy fantasizing during sex about being raped, but there isn't a single woman who actually desires that.

• **Don't confuse politics with clinical/pastoral work.**

For example, you may be concerned that people who consume pornography are motivated to commit violence against women (although as we've already seen, the data generally refutes this concern). Unless you think your current client is particularly vulnerable to such a motivation, your concern about "men" would be irrelevant regarding his case. The same is true about any concerns you have about "men" supporting an industry that you consider unsavory or even involved with human trafficking (again, the data refutes this concern). That's a political, not a clinical consideration, and it's inappropriate for you to discourage a client from using porn because of it.

• **If appropriate, do raise your clients' porn literacy.**

Sometimes a porn consumer and/or his partner will benefit from their increased literacy regarding porn. Part of that is challenging people about the myths we've already discussed. It also includes making sure clients know:

~ Porn isn't a documentary; real sex and real bodies aren't like that.
~ Real sex doesn't *feel* the way porn *looks.*
~ Porn omits parts of sex that most people consider important, including kissing, embracing, talking, laughing, and contraception.
~ A sexual encounter in real life almost never starts the way it begins in porn. It generally requires conversation, a smile, and a gentle touch.
~ Without scripting and a lot of preparation, much of what takes place in porn would be very uncomfortable, extremely unlikely, or simply impossible.
~ Most people never do some of the commonest things in porn: ejaculating on a woman's face; anal sex; threesomes; women squirting during orgasm; sex with strangers; same-gender sex to orgasm. There isn't anything wrong with these, but porn makes them seem common, and they are actually very unusual in the general population.

• **Don't assume that if you get a man to use less porn, he'll have more desire for his wife or girlfriend.**

This is like assuming that if someone eats less ice cream, they'll eat more broccoli. If a man wants to increase his desire for his partner, techniques include focusing on the parts of her that he finds attractive, speaking with her about specific activities, addressing contraception, discovering and repairing old resentments or wounds, and improving their relationship. Most of all, we'd want to find out what has reduced his desire for her (if he ever had any), and the extent to which he has desire for anyone.

When masturbation is a form of self-soothing, or reassurance of function, or an experience of autonomy, taking it away hardly helps to enhance a relationship with a partner.

• **Remember that for some people, what looks like overinvolvement with porn is actually overinvolvement with the Internet.**

We're all still learning how to cope with the Internet's unlimited hunting opportunities, the unheard-of variety of images of whatever we're interested in (puppies, movie stars, lasagna), and the fact that this extraordinary picture-and-word contraption is available for both work and play. In fact, many people's lifestyle has completely blurred the distinction between work and play. One man's lost-in-porn is another man's (or woman's) lost-in-Disney memorabilia or compulsive *Downton Abbey* sneak-watching in between customers.

• **Remember that adult porn is *not* a gateway to, or the same as, child porn.**

America's porn industry is a multi-billion dollar enterprise marketing a legal product. They have no interest in expanding into a profoundly illegal market niche that everyone knows will get you bankrupt, jailed, and brutalized.

Everyone acting in American commercial porn must be certified as 18 and older. People who like to look at porn featuring young-looking actresses know they're looking at adults, even though they may like pretending they're looking at high school students. There is no evidence that such fantasy viewing leads to a demand for highly illegal, elusive, and obscure porn featuring actual minors.

• **Therapists, social workers, clergy: Remember that *your* profession is in the grip of a PornPanic, too.**

This means your training in pornography is probably limited or even misinformed; it probably includes a political correctness that limits dissenting voices with actual data or alternative counseling approaches; you face a mass media and public demanding that you compromise your professional principles to deal with their fear, anger, and confusion; and you face clients who are highly emotional about the subject, frightened for their family, and possibly overreacting to events in their lives.

• **If you're going to counsel people about parenting around porn, you need to know what kids do around it.**

If you're interested, go to websites that serve kids' needs around sexual information. You may be surprised at the frankness with which kids are discussing sex and with which educators are responding to them. You'll probably be surprised at the sophistication with which young people navigate websites, social media, and their own devices when it comes to porn, sexting, and pursuing information.

Great websites in this regard are Scarleteen; Sex, etc.; SIECUS; and Laci Green's video blog, *Sex Plus.*

• You need a definition of healthy porn use.

If you don't have one and don't want one, you're probably not prepared to deal with cases in which pornography is an issue. It's up to the client to decide whether he wants to discontinue using pornography, not you.

• Remember that just because a case involves porn there isn't necessarily a porn problem. Here are examples of cases that include porn which are about much more than porn:

~ He pressures his wife to watch porn with him, although she doesn't want to.
~ He demands his girlfriend do what he sees women do in porn.
~ She feels obliged to do what he demands.
~ He leaves evidence of his masturbation around the house despite the fact that (or perhaps because) she resents him masturbating.
~ She tells him she understands why he watches porn better than he does.
~ He carelessly leaves porn on his computer or device so that his kids stumble onto it.
~ He makes rude jokes about porn in the family or in public.
~ He spends rent money on porn.
~ They argue periodically about whether or not he's "allowed" to watch porn.
~ He's promised to stop watching porn, and then she catches him doing it and resents it.
~ She makes snide comments about porn whenever a TV show or the news gives her the opportunity.
~ She withdraws (emotionally and/or sexually) from her husband in disgust over his porn viewing.
~ She talks critically to her kids about her husband's or ex-husband's porn viewing.

These are all examples of dysfunctional and irresponsible behaviors that happen to involve porn—but they could be about almost anything and look the same. For example, pressuring someone to watch football games on TV when they clearly dislike doing so; spending the rent money on fishing equipment or new sweaters; carelessly leaving sharp knives or valuables around where kids could hurt themselves or the family.

What may present as porn cases are often cases about power, responsibility, passive-aggressiveness, retaliation, existential loneliness, fear of growing old, etc. Look for those themes rather than getting distracted by the porn elements of a case.

• Do encourage couples to discuss sex more than pornography.

As I've said throughout this book, many couples with sexual difficulties find it almost impossible to discuss them with each other. Common difficulties include desire discrepancies; lack of orgasm or satisfaction; low frequency; conflict about preferences; infidelity; suspicion of infidelity (which is not the same thing as infidelity); problems with arousal or excitement; and the incredibly common situation of little or no sex in long-term relationships.

Pornography is an easy thing for couples to fight about, as it can involve issues of power, fantasy, violence, fear, arousal, gender, desire, masturbation, attraction, autonomy, dysfunction, rejection, and self-esteem, all without leaving the comfort of your own home. You might want to assess which of these any given client(s) really needs to discuss before delving into pornography.

EPILOGUE: A COMPLICATED CONSUMER PRODUCT

Because of our tormented relationship with sexuality, America loads a lot of things onto pornography. We blame it for the results of how we raise our kids, run our marriages, advertise consumer products, and make sexual decisions. We disapprove of the results of what we do, and then we blame porn for these results. Not only is this intellectually dishonest, it keeps us stuck getting what we don't want. Because porn isn't going away, our investment in blaming porn for what we fear, hate, and feel ashamed of guarantees more fear, more hate, and more shame.

The PornPanic enterprise most certainly makes our lives worse. As I said almost 10 years ago in *America's War on Sex*, there's an unlimited amount of money and power to be gained by scaring the hell out of Americans about sex. This is true regarding porn. And as we've seen in Part I, with the transition from the "immorality" problem to the "public health/danger" problem, more and more groups are jumping on the anti-porn bandwagon, making the PornPanic more intense and more frightening than ever.

These groups include anti-trafficking activists; anti-sex work abolitionists; Internet safety advocates; child safety advocates; radical feminists; religious leaders; anti-masturbation crusaders; sexual purity crusaders; conservative women's political groups; politicians; anti-domestic violence activists; and people who make a living "treating" porn addiction.

Alternately cynical and naïve, the combined PornPanic enterprises actively promote gossip, rumors, and recycled junk "statistics" to show that porn is dangerous for not just its users, but for everyone else, too. Ironically, it's some of these same groups that lobby against funding the science that could establish the actual impacts of porn. This is similar to the way the gun lobby has successfully helped Congress prevent government funding of public health research that could definitively answer questions about whether guns are dangerous—and then the gun lobby says, "There's no proof that guns are dangerous."

I don't know anyone who uses porn who says, "We shouldn't have research about porn's effects." But a lot of people who say that porn is dangerous lobby against scientifically researching porn's effects. They counter the federal research of the 1960s, 1970s, and 1980s that found no harm from porn by saying "today's porn is different"—but then they block today's scientists from studying today's porn. (This is also the reason we lack sufficient data on the effects of viewing child pornography.)

By preventing research on the effects of porn, endlessly repeating Big Lies about porn's effects, and simultaneously opposing sex education that addresses pornography honestly, the PornPanic perpetuates the problems we so much lament and fear. Because we don't properly educate our kids about sex, don't train health or mental health professionals in porn and how it's used, and don't have honest discussions about the uses of sexuality in advertising and the arts, we get to blame porn for a lot—and solve nothing.

In this regime, the enemy is clear, the only solution is increased ignorance, and the result devoutly wished is a narrowed scope of human sexual imagination.

This outcome will not happen. Instead, the opposite will: more porn, more confusion, more rancorous struggles on all sides, more attempts at censorship, and more marital strife. That's the bitter harvest of PornPanic.

It's interesting, however, to note the obsessive focus on negative outcomes of porn use. For obvious political and ideological reasons, there is little call for research (or even discussion) about possible positive outcomes of porn use. These positive outcomes might include:

Facilitate dialog with a partner
Get new ideas for erotic activities (costumes, positions, dialog)
Prevent/relieve boredom in long-term relationships
Endorse female sexual desire, agency, and pleasure
Normalize masturbation
Educate about female sexual anatomy
Model behaviors such as outercourse (non-intercourse sex)

The lack of this side of the conversation about pornography is telling. It tells us that the anti-porn crusade is about something other than porn, and that its agendas are about more than preventing negative outcomes. There's a clear anti-sex agenda, often an anti-female sexuality agenda.

Many products in everyday use can be exploitative or dangerous, including cars, alcohol, Viagra, fireworks, smartphones, rock 'n' roll, tattoos, and even ibuprofen.

The positives of such products are always raised when their negative aspects are discussed. This is even true of professional football, a wildly popular product now fighting to control its public image and maintain its customer base. Whenever concussions or CTE are discussed, NFL spokespersons don't deny football is dangerous, but contextualize this fact within a values statement that "yes, but all life involves risk, and football offers millions of participants and spectators a lot of good things."[1]

Those responding to the common one-sided, negative view of pornography, by contrast, generally use unsophisticated, ineffectual arguments:

1. No, porn isn't dangerous, or
2. It doesn't matter if it is, because America's tradition of free expression mandates porn's availability, and consumers have a right to access this content.

While the first is mostly true and the second is entirely true, this is simply not sufficient. In today's America (as in yesterday's), consumers aren't willing to stand up on behalf of this product, and its creators similarly feel blocked from advocating for its positives. Scientists aren't studying it. The media are caught in the very PornPanic they're supposed to be reporting on, so it's almost impossible for them to see through it clearly enough to describe it and its typical effects accurately.

And when people hypothesize this product's unique negative impacts—such as badly educating young people or modeling disrespect to women—we should wonder why these critics aren't in favor of public policies and social norms that would influence these issues about which they apparently care so much. Comprehensive sex education, more parent–child conversations about sex, better training of clinicians, a more fair and accurate media narrative, and new norms about how couples can talk about sexuality would be a good start.

In fact, a sufficient amount of the above would resolve most problems about pornography. As I've been describing throughout this book, the best approach to America's destructive PornPanic is honest talk about sex. And lots of it.

NOTES

INTRODUCTION

1. The adaptation of new technologies for sexual purposes: Pottery: Used as a medium for erotic art; Gutenberg: Some of the first books printed with the new movable type were erotic manuscripts; Rubber: Used for a new kind of condom; Nylon: Used for a new kind of hosiery.

2. The question was repeated by a government prosecutor in the British obscenity trial of *Lady Chatterley's Lover*. See http://ahr.oxfordjournals.org/content/118/3/653.full.html

3. Even as the public (1) has made Internet pornography one of the most popular forms of entertainment in history, and (2) has made the Internet the cornerstone of all private, public, and commercial interactions with blinding speed.

4. ArmyTimes.com, http://www.armytimes.com/article/20100331/OFFDUTY03/3310301/Addicted-online-porn

5. DailyMail.co.uk, http://www.dailymail.co.uk/news/article-2261377/Porn-study-scrapped-researchers-failed-ANY-20-males-hadn-t-watched-it.html

CHAPTER ONE

1. Archive.org, https://archive.org/details/Perversi1965

2. Prochoice.org, http://prochoice.org/education-and-advocacy/violence/violence-statistics-and-history

3. A term introduced by the Family Research Council in 1992, https://en.wikipedia.org/wiki/Homosexual_agenda#Initial_usage

4. More than 17,000 people allege that Catholic priests were sexual with them as children. Allegations against more than 6,000 priests are deemed "credible." BishopAccountability.org, http://www.bishop-accountability.org/AtAGlance /USCCB_Yearly_Data_on_Accused_Priests.htm

5. Oyez.org, https://www.oyez.org/cases/2002/02-102

6. Kennedy said that the Constitution protects "personal decisions relating to marriage, procreation, contraception, family relationships, [and] child rearing" and that homosexuals "may seek autonomy for these purposes." The Court held that "the Texas statute furthers no legitimate state interest which can justify its intrusion into the personal and private life of the individual." In his scathing dissent, Scalia described the decision as ". . . the Court asserts [that] the promotion of majoritarian sexual morality is not even a *legitimate* state interest. . . ." Law .Cornell.edu, https://www.law.cornell.edu/supct/html/02-102.ZD.html

7. Oyez.org, https://www.oyez.org/cases/1985/85-140

8. Contrast this with the United Kingdom, whose tabloids like *The Sun* featured nude women on Page 3 each day.

9. The government soon outlawed such naughty postcards.

10. See *America's War on Sex: The Continuing Attack on Law, Lust, and Liberty.* Santa Barbara, CA: Praeger Publishers, 2006, Chapter 2.

11. See *America's War on Sex*, sidebar, page 39.

12. For the most comprehensive information about Internet filtering (or "blocking") software, see www.peacefire.org.

13. Alternet.org, http://www.alternet.org/sex-amp-relationships/10-craziest -ways-sex-has-changed

CHAPTER TWO

1. I have been writing about sexual moral panics for decades; see *America's War on Sex*, my articles for *Playboy*, my articles on sex addiction, and my blog at https://sexualintelligence.wordpress.com.

Others who have written extensively on sexuality-related moral panics in America include Stanley Cohen, Mickey Diamond, Paula Fass, Gil Herdt, Dagmar Herzog, Laura Kipnis, James Morone, and Dan Savage.

2. Gil Herdt, ed., *Moral Panics, Sex Panics: Fear and the Fight over Sexual Rights.* New York: New York University Press, 2009.

3. Discussed in David Hajdu, *The Ten-Cent Plague: The Great Comic-Book Scare and How It Changed America.* London: Picador Press, 2009.

4. TheComicBooks.com, http://www.thecomicbooks.com/1954senatetran scripts.html

5. Advocate.com, http://www.advocate.com/politics/2014/07/25/michele -bachmann-back-one-her-most-homophobic-comments-ever

6. RightWingWatch.org, http://www.rightwingwatch.org/content/bach mann-god-may-destroy-america-over-gay-marriage-just-sodom

7. *JAMA Pediatrics*; see UNH.edu, http://www.unh.edu/ccrc/pdf/poil 30100.pdf. See also FreeRangeKids.com, http://www.freerangekids.com/crime -statistics/

8. At least 25 percent of America's registered sex offenders are minors. A substantial percentage of all registered sex offenders were convicted of non-contact offenses, such as voyeurism, exhibitionism, and teen sexting. Registered sex offenders have trouble getting jobs, loans, and often have to move out of their homes because they're located too close to churches, schools, or bus stops—or because they live in a house with a sibling under 18 years old.

The Adam Walsh Child Safety Protection Act of 2006 requires states to put juveniles over the age of 14 on public sex offender registries if they (a) commit a sex offense equivalent to or worse than aggravated sexual assault against a victim under the age of 12, or (b) commit any sex-related offense for which they were tried and convicted as an adult.

9. ClassicBands.com, http://www.classicbands.com/banned.html

10. Alfred C Kinsey, Wardell Baxter Pomeroy and Clyde E Martin, *Sexual Behavior in the Human Male.* Philadelphia: W.B. Saunders Co., 1948. Led by monomaniacal Judith Reisman, right-wing and conspiracy-type websites still blame Kinsey's work as the cause of today's alleged sexual immorality. The title of Reisman's bizarre book on Kinsey says it all: *Sexual Sabotage: How One Mad Scientist Unleashed a Plague of Corruption and Contagion on America.* Los Angeles: WND Books, 2010.

11. "As early as 1744, Northampton minister Jonathan Edwards initiated a church inquiry into the 'lascivious expressions' of certain young men who had read the Master-Piece and had taunted local women with their newly acquired 'unclean' knowledge of female anatomy contained in it." GerardKoeppel.com, http://gerardkoeppel.com/wp-content/uploads/2015/10/enan_eriecanal.pdf

12. Google.com, https://www.google.com/webhp?sourceid=chrome-instant &ion=1&espv=2&ie=UTF-8#q=how+many+internet+users+in+US+in+1999

InternetLiveStates.com, http://www.internetlivestats.com/internet-users /united-states

13. People recently had another lesson about that in 2015 with the Ashley Madison hacking scandal. People were shocked that a corporation might actually lie about the way it handled their private data. See Fortune.com, http:// fortune.com/2015/08/26/ashley-madison-hack

14. K9WebProtection.com, www.k9webprotection.com

15. For more on the inadequacies of these filtering products and outright deception of these filtering companies, see www.peacefire.org.

16. For a colorful account of how one such extortion site was successfully sued, see Randazza.Wordpress.com, https://randazza.wordpress.com/2014/03 /18/revenge-porn-scumbags-spanked-with-385000-judgment.

CHAPTER THREE

1. Even churches and religious groups, while noting how offended God is by porn, are now quick to note that porn also leads to divorce, destroys families, endangers children, etc. Their dual approach (never mention porn's immorality without also mentioning its dangers) is like the extra safety provided by wearing suspenders and a belt.

2. PureIntimacy.org, http://www.pureintimacy.org/f/fatal-addiction-ted
-bundys-final-interview/

3. Rense.com, http://www.rense.com/general86/porno.htm

4. (Pronounced "public-eyesd") For a discussion of this see *America's War
on Sex*, p. 172.

5. Note that porn consumers have not organized themselves into a stakeholder
group.

6. Dines argues that using dildos or vibrators turns women into sexual
objects (Dines, G. "Dirty Business: *Playboy Magazine* and the Mainstreaming
of Pornography," p. 61); Russo objects to porn's focus on pleasure, which suggests that sex is about "individual self-fulfillment" when it should be about
"social change" (Russo, A. "Feminists Confront Pornography's Subordinating
Practices: Policies and Strategies for Change," p. 34); Jensen and Dines object to
images of enthusiastic sex, as they convey the message that men don't have to
work at giving women sexual pleasure, p. 72. These references are all in Jensen
and Dines (eds.), *Pornography: The Production and Consumption of Inequality*.
New York: Routledge, 1998.

7. Recurring sources for inaccurate myths about porn include Phil Burress, Gail
Dines, Andrea Dworkin, Sue Johnson, Mary Anne Layden, Catharine MacKinnon, Penny Nance, Judith Reisman, Pat Robertson, and Marnia Robinson.

8. *Hollywood Reporter*, http://www.hollywoodreporter.com/news/fifty
-shades-grey-sales-hit-683852

9. *Huffington* Post, http://www.huffingtonpost.com/2012/07/25/half-of
-americans-drink-soda-everyday-consumption_n_1699540.html

INTERLUDE A:
THE NATURE OF SEXUAL FANTASY

1. Ogi Ogas and Sai Gaddam, *A Billion Wicked Thoughts*. New York: Pen-
guin, 2011.

2. Suzanne Sarnoff and Irving Sarnoff, *Masturbation and Adult Sexuality*.
New York: Evans & Co., 1979.

3. Pornhub.com, http://www.pornhub.com/insights/united-states-top
-searches http://www.pornhub.com/insights/2014-year-in-review

INTERLUDE B:
DEEP IN THE VALLEY: GOING TO A PORN SHOOT

1. Barbara Nitke, *American Ecstasy*. New York: Pierrot Press, 2012.

INTERLUDE E:
NO, MABEL, YOU DON'T HAVE TO COMPETE
WITH PORN ACTRESSES

1. Viralscape.com, http://viralscape.com/supermodels-without-makeup/

CHAPTER FIVE

1. KnopfDoubleday.com, http://knopfdoubleday.com/2011/03/14/your-cell-phone

2. Originating around 1970, Moore's Law states that computer processing power will double every two years. See MooresLaw.org, www.mooreslaw.org.

3. Kaitlin Lounsbury, Kimberly Mitchell, and David Finkelhor, "The True Prevalence of 'Sexting'," in bulletin of Crimes Against Children Research Center, April 2011.

4. Kimberly Mitchell, Lisa Jones, David Finkelhor, and Janis Wolak, "Youth Involvement in Sexting: Findings from the Youth Internet Safety Studies" in bulletin of Crimes Against Children Research Center, February 2014.

5. Hanna Rosin, *The Atlantic*, http://www.theatlantic.com/magazine/archive/2014/11/why-kids-sext/380798/

6. Wikipedia.org, https://en.wikipedia.org/wiki/Ages_of_consent_in_the_United_States

7. Hanna Rosin, *The Atlantic*, http://www.theatlantic.com/magazine/archive/2014/11/why-kids-sext/380798/

8. AmyHasinoff.Wordpress.com, https://amyhasinoff.wordpress.com/book/

9. AmyHasinoff.Wordpress.com, https://amyhasinoff.wordpress.com/book/

10. Janis Wolak and David Finkelhor, "Sexting: A Typology," in bulletin of Crimes Against Children Research Center, March 2011. http://www.unh.edu/ccrc/pdf/CV231_Sexting%20Typology%20Bulletin_4-6-11_revised.pdf

11. For a list and synopses of young adult fiction with nuanced depictions of sexual consent, see http://www.teenlibrariantoolbox.com/2014/03/take-5-sexconsent-positive-books-the-svyalit-project/

12. Peggy Orenstein, *Girls and Sex: Navigating the Complicated New Landscape*. New York, NY: Harper, 2016.

13. Time.com, http://time.com/4103885/massive-sexting-ring-stuns-colorado-high-school/

14. *The Atlantic*, http://www.theatlantic.com/magazine/archive/2014/11/why-kids-sext/380798/

15. *The Atlantic*, http://www.theatlantic.com/magazine/archive/2014/11/why-kids-sext/380798

16. Link.Springer.com, http://link.springer.com/article/10.1007/s13178-014-0162-9

17. *The Atlantic*, http://www.theatlantic.com/magazine/archive/2014/11/why-kids-sext/380798/

18. Number of Americans arrested for a marijuana possession in 2013: 609,423. Number of students who have lost federal financial aid eligibility because of a drug conviction: 200,000+. DrugPolicy.org, http://www.drugpolicy.org/drug-war-statistics

19. PsychologyToday.com, https://www.psychologytoday.com/blog/teen-angst/201308/teens-who-click-send-and-sext

20. For the laws that govern underage sexting in each state, see IM.About .com, http://im.about.com/od/sexting. Of course, the site's accuracy cannot be guaranteed.

CHAPTER SIX

1. Matthew 5:28, Proverbs 6:25, James 1:14–15, 1 Corinthians 6:18–20.

CASE A: RACHEL & JACKSON

1. This recalls the joke about the parishioner who is warned about this exact point as he completes confession. On his way out of church, he pauses at the collection box, then continues toward the exit. When the priest calls out, "You forgot to put a donation in the box," the parishioner replies, "That's OK, I thought about it."

CHAPTER SEVEN

1. Ronald Weitzer, "Review Essay: Pornography's Effects: The Need for Solid Evidence." *Violence Against Women*, 2011. 17:666. Originally published online April 21, 2011. DI: 10.1177/1077801211407478.

2. Johnson, Eithne, "Appearing Live on Your Campus!: Porn-education roadshows," *Jump Cut*, 41, 1997, pp.27–35.

3. "For many perpetrators, there is a progression from viewing adult pornography to viewing child pornography." "If we tolerate pornographic material that encourages people to indulge their darkest sexual fantasies, we cannot act surprised when millions do so in real life as well." MoralityInMedia.org, http://moralityin media.org/full_article.php?article_no=45

4. Daniel Weiss, "Porn Feeds Human Trafficking," DenverPost.com, 1/27/2006.

5. Susan Brownmiller, *Against Our Will: Men, Women and Rape*. New York: Fawcett Columbine, 1993 (1975).

6. R. Jensen, Introduction. In G. Dines R. Jensen, and A. Russo (eds.), *Pornography: The Production and Consumption of Inequality*. New York: Rutledge, 1997.

7. E. Donnerstein, and L. Berkowitz, "Victim Reactions in Aggressive Erotic Films as a Factor in Violence Against Women." *Journal of Personality and Social Psychology*, 1981. 41:4, 710–24.

8. William Fisher and G. Grenier, "Violent Pornography, Anti-Woman Thoughts and Anti-Woman Acts: In Search of Reliable Effects." *Journal of Sex Research*, 1994. 31, 23–38.

9. BJS.gov, http://www.bjs.gov/content/pub/pdf/rsavcaf9513.pdf

10. Gail Dines, *Pornland: How Porn Has Hijacked Our Sexuality*. Boston: Beacon, 2010.

11. R. Jensen, "Pornography Is What the End of the World Looks Like," in Karen Boyle, ed., *Everyday Pornography*. New York: Routledge, 2010.

12. Comedians who have used rape jokes in their acts and discussed reactions to them (including intense online attacks) include Sarah Silverman, Louis CK, Daniel Tosh, Chris Rock, and Jimmy Carr.

13. Anthony D'Amato, "Porn Up, Rape Down." Public Law and Legal Theory Research Paper Series, 2006. Retrieved 3/23/16 from http://anthonydamato .law.northwestern.edu/Adobefiles/porn.pdf

14. NIJ.gov, http://www.nij.gov/journals/254/pages/rape_reporting.aspx. In fact, the rate at which women report rape and attempted rape has actually gone up. Thus if the reported rape rate has gone down, that represents an improvement bigger than just the difference between the rate now and the rate before.

15. G. Dines, R. Jensen, and A. Russo, *Pornography: The Production and Consumption of Inequality.* New York: Routledge, 1997.

16. Neil M. Malamuth, Tamara Addison, and Mary Koss, "Pornography and Sexual Aggression: Are There Reliable Effects and Can We Understand Them?" doi: 10.1080/10532528.2000.10559784 pp 26–91. *Annual Review of Sex Research*, Vol. 11 Issue 1, 2000.

17. D.A. Kingston et al., "The Importance of Individual Differences in Pornography Use: Theoretical Perspectives and Implications of Treating Sexual Offenders." *Journal of Sex Research*, 2009. 46(203), 216–232. Doi:10.1080/00224490902747701

18. Michael Seto, Alexandra Maric, and Howard Barbaree, "The Role of Pornography in the Etiology of Sexual Aggression." *Aggression and Violent Behavior*, Vol. 6, Issue 1, Jan-Feb 2001, pp. 35–53.

19. Cindy M. Meston, and Lucia F. O'Sullivan, "Such a Tease: Intentional Sexual Provocation within Heterosexual Interactions," 2007. *Archives of Sexual Behavior*, 36:531–542. doi 10.1007/s10508-006-9167-7.

20. Rebecca Whisnant, Essay in Karen Boyle, ed. *Everyday Pornography.* New York: Routledge, 2010, pp. 114, 115.

21. Gail Dines, *Pornland: How Porn Has Hijacked Our Sexuality.* Boston: Beacon, 2010, p. xvii.

22. Ana Bridges, Essay in Karen Boyle, ed., *Everyday Pornography.* New York: Routledge, 2010, p. 47.

23. Meagan Tyler, essay in Karen Boyle, ed., *Everyday Pornography.* New York: Routledge, 2010, p. 57.

24. R.E. Funk, "What Does Pornography Say about Me(n)?" In Stark, C. and Whisnant, R. (eds.), *Not for Sale: Feminists Resisting Prostitution and Pornography*, Melbourne, Australia: Spinifex Press, p. 341.

25. R. Jensen, R and G. Dines, "The Content of Mass Marketed Pornography." In G. Dines, R. Jensen, and A. Russo, *Pornography: The Production and Consumption of Inequality.* New York: Routledge, 1997, pp. 76, 83.

26. Hawaii.edu, http://www.hawaii.edu/PCSS/biblio/articles/2005to2009 /2009-pornography-acceptance-crime.html

27. Alan McKee, "The Aesthetics of Pornography: The Insights of Consumers," *Journal of Media & Cultural Studies*, Vol. 20, No. 4, December 2006, pp. 523–39.

28. F. Attwood, "'Other' or 'One of Us'?: The Porn User in Public and Academic Discourse," *Participations: Journal of Audience and Reception Studies*, 2007, 4 (1).

29. J.M. Albright, "Sex in America Online: An Exploration of Sex, Marital Status, and Sexual Identity in Internet Sex Seeking and Its Impacts." *Journal of Sex Research*, 2008, 45(2), 175–186. http://dx.doi.org/10.1080/002244980 1987481. Medline: 18569538.

Bridges, Bergner, and Hesson-McInnes, "Romantic Partners' Use of Pornography: Its Significance for Women." *Journal of Sex & Marital Therapy*, 2003, 29(1), 1–14. http://dx.doi.org/10.1080/713847097 Medline 12519658

G.M. Hald and N.M. Malamuth, "Self-Perceived Effects of Pornography Consumption," *Archives of Sexual Behavior*, 2008, 37(4), 614–625. http://dx.doi.org/10.1007/210508-007-9212-1 Medline 17851749

M.A. Watson and R.D. Smith. "Positive Porn: Educational, Medical, and Clinical Uses," *Am J Sex Educ.* 2012;7(2):122–45. doi:10.1080/15546128.2012.680861.

Alan McKee. "The Positive and Negative Effects of Pornography as Attributed by Consumers." *Aust J Commun.* 2007; 34(1):87–104.

30. A. Štulhofer, V. Buško, and I. Landripet. "Pornography, Sexual Socialization, and Satisfaction among Young Men," *Arch Sex Behav.* 2010;39(1):168–78. doi:10.1007/s10508-008-9387-0.

Alan McKee, "The Need to Bring the Voices of Pornography Consumers into Public Debates about the Genre and Its Effects," *Australian Journal of Communication* 32(2), 2005, pp. 71–94.

Alan McKee, "The Relationship Between Attitudes Towards Women, Consumption of Pornography, and Other Demographic Variables in a Survey of 1023 Consumers of Pornography," *Journal of Psychology and Human Sexuality*, 18(2), 2006.

Alan McKee, "Censorship of Sexually Explicit Materials in Australia: What Do Consumers of Pornography Have to Say About It?," *Media International Australia*, 120, 2006, pp. 35–50.

Alan McKee, "The Aesthetics of Pornography: The Insights of Consumers," *Continuum: Journal of Media and Cultural Studies*, 20, 2006, pp. 523–439.

31. C. Staley and N. Prause, "Erotica Viewing Effects on Intimate Relationships and Self/Partner Evaluations," *Archives of Sexual Behavior*, 2013, 42(4), 615–624. http://dx.doi.org/10.1017/s10508-012-0034-4 Medline:23224749.

32. R. Jensen and G. Dines, "The Content of Mass Marketed Pornography." In G. Dines, R. Jensen, and A. Russo, *Pornography: The Production and Consumption of Inequality.* New York: Routledge, 1997, p. 163.

33. Taylor Kohut and Jodie Baer, "Is Pornography Really about Making Hate to Women? Pornography Users Hold More Gender Egalitarian Attitudes Than Nonusers in a Representative American Sample," *Journal of Sex Research*, 2016, 53(1), 1–11.

34. GailDines.com, http://gaildines.com/2009/09/so-you-think-you-know-what-porn-is/ para. 25.

35. D. Loftus, *Watching Sex: How Men Really Respond to Pornography*. New York: Thunder's Mouth, 2002.

CHAPTER EIGHT

1. WebMD.com, http://www.webmd.com/balance/guide/addicted-your-smartphone-what-to-do

2. NoozHawk.com, http://www.noozhawk.com/article/092210_russell_collins_the_puzzling_problem_of_internet_porn

ScholarsArchive.BYE.edu, http://scholarsarchive.byu.edu/cgi/viewcontent.cgi?article=4081&context=etd

LucilleZimmerman.com, http://www.lucillezimmerman.com/2012/09/27/the-cure-for-sexual-addiction-is-attachment

PsychOfMen.Wordpress.com, https://psychofmen.wordpress.com/final-papers/the-study-of-men-and-sexual-addictions

3. This is similar to the high levels of superstition among accomplished athletes—a reaction to the unpredictable nature of elite performance. See Psychology OfSports.com, http://psychologyofsports.com/2004/06/23/superstition-in-sports-2

CHAPTER NINE

1. Universally accepted diagnostic criteria do not exist for pornography addiction or problematic pornography viewing. See M.P. Twohig and J.M. Crosby, "Acceptance and Commitment Therapy as a Treatment for Problematic Internet Pornography Viewing," *Behavior Therapy*, 2010, 41 (3): 285–295. doi:10.1016/j.beth.2009.06.002.PMID 20569778.

2. In fact, in some programs "porn addicts" are even told that they have to abstain from partner sex for awhile.

3. Patrick Carnes, *Out of the Shadows: Understanding Sexual Addiction*. Minneapolis: CompCare Publishers, 1983.

4. Because there are no agreed-upon, peer-reviewed diagnostic criteria, the incidence of "sex addiction" is debatable. Some common estimates—whose criteria are not published—are:

Patrick Carnes: 5–8 percent of the adult public;

Rob Weiss: 3–5 percent of the adult public;

Mayo Clinic: 3–6 percent of the adult public.

5. For the APA's own description on the extensive revision process, see DSM5.org, http://www.dsm5.org/about/pages/faq.aspx

6. "Viewing online pornography" is specifically mentioned. APA.org, http://www.apa.org/monitor/2014/04/pornography.aspx

Slate.com, http://www.slate.com/blogs/xx_factor/2015/08/27/josh_duggar_is_going_to_rehab_for_porn_addiction_is_that_a_real_thing.html

NCBI.NLM.NIH,gov, http://www.ncbi.nlm.nih.gov/pmc/articles/PMC4600144

https://en.wikipedia.org/wiki/Pornography_addiction#cite_note-twohig 2010-5

7. UPI.com, http://www.upi.com/Health_News/2014/02/12/Researchers -No-such-thing-as-porn-addiction/UPI-84311392244818/#ixzz2tDtPg8UD

8. "I was a porn addict and now I can help you." See CompulsionSolutions .com, http://compulsionsolutions.com

9. A lot of what looks like porn addiction to some is certainly a matter of the social or psychological environment in which a person is located. See Michael W. Ross, Sven-Axel Månsson, Kristian Daneback, "Prevalence, Severity, and Correlates of Problematic Sexual Internet Use in Swedish Men and Women." *Archives of Sexual Behavior*, April 2012, Vol. 41, Issue 2 pp. 459–466. First online: 12 May 2011. doi:10.1007/s10508-011-9762-0

10. Cancer.org, http://www.cancer.org/healthy/stayawayfromtobacco/guide toquittingsmoking/guide-to-quitting-smoking-success-rates

11. DailyMail.co.uk, http://www.dailymail.co.uk/health/article-2292468 /Average-smoker-makes-failed-attempts-habit-finally-so.html#ixzz3xGf92jO3

12. DrOz.com, http://www.doctoroz.com/videos/can-porn-cause-erectile -dysfunction-pt-1

13. Personal communication, Charles Moser, MD.

14. N. Prause and J. Pfaus, "Viewing Sexual Stimuli Associated with Greater Sexual Responsiveness, Not Erectile Dysfunction." *Sex Med* 2015. doi:10.1002/ sm2.58 [epub ahead of print]

15. I. Landripet and A. Stulhofer, "Is Pornography Use Associated with Sexual Difficulties and Dysfunctions among Younger Heterosexual Men?" *Journal of Sex Medicine*, 2015; 12:1136–1139.

16. WebMD.com, http://www.webmd.com/erectile-dysfunction/news/200 40804/young-men-lead-surge-in-viagra-use

17. One reason physicians mistakenly think they are seeing more ED in young men is because some patients want erection drugs for performance enhancement rather than real ED, and they know what to say to get them. See the study on faked ADHD and Adderall seeking: M. Sollman, "Detection of Feigned ADHD in College Students," *Psychological Assessment* 2010 Vol. 22, No. 2, 325–335. "Results indicated malingerers readily produced ADHD-consistent profiles."

18. In her APS-David Myers Distinguished Lecture on the Science and Craft of Teaching Psychology, 5/25/12. PsychologicalScience.org, http://www .psychologicalscience.org/index.php/video/how-to-spot-pseudoneuroscience -and-biobunk.html 13:15-13:45 slide.

19. D.P. McCabe and A.D. Castel, Department of Psychology at Colorado State University, "Seeing is Believing: The Effect of Brain Images on Judgments of Scientific Reasoning," *Cognition* 2008, Apr;107(1):343–52. Epub Sept. 4, 2007.

20. Salon.com, http://www.salon.com/2012/03/20/santorums_bad_porn _science

21. Salon.com, http://www.salon.com/2012/03/20/santorums_bad_porn _science

22. Salon.com, http://www.salon.com/2012/03/20/santorums_bad_porn _science

23. Independent.co.uk, http://www.independent.co.uk/life-style/health-and -families/health-news/pornography-addiction-leads-to-same-brain-activity-as -alcoholism-or-drug-abuse-study-shows-8832708.html

24. Personal communication, 9/23/13.

25. SmithsonianMag.com, http://www.smithsonianmag.com/smart-news /the-smell-of-newborn-babies-triggers-the-same-reward-centers-as-drugs -58482/?no-ist

26. J.R. Georgiadis and M.L. Kringelbach. "The Human Sexual Response Cycle: Brain Imaging Evidence Linking Sex to Other Pleasures," *Prog Neurobiol.* 2012; 98(1):49–81. doi:10.1016/j.pneurobio.2012.05.004.

27. J.R. Georgiadis, "Regional Cerebral Blood Flow Changes Associated with Clitorally Induced Orgasm in Healthy Women," *European Journal of Neuroscience*, 2006, *24*(11), 3305–3316.

28. YourBrainOnPorn.com, http://yourbrainonporn.com/ask-us-iam-attra cted-to-gay-transsexual

29. Paula Hall, *Understanding and Treating Sex Addiction: A Comprehensive Guide for People Who Struggle with Sex Addiction and Those Who Want to Help Them.* New York: Routledge, 2012.

30. P.A. Trueman, "Porn Creates Demand for Sex Trafficking." *Miami Herald* [online] July 2. 2014. http://www.miamiherald.com/2014/07/23/4251372 /porn-creates-demand-for-sex-trafficking.html

Of course, there is only a tiny amount of sex trafficking in the United States at the very same time that there is a huge amount of porn consumption.

31. NoFap.com, http://www.nofap.com

32. Sydney.edu.au, http://sydney.edu.au/news/84.html?newsstoryid=9176

EPILOGUE

1. See NFL Commissioner Roger Goodell's statements in the *New York Times Magazine*, 2/7/16, and *San Jose Mercury-News*, 2/6/16.

INDEX

Abstinence model, 13, 95
Adam Walsh Child Safety Protection
    Act of 2006, 191n8
Adams, Abigail, 40
Adaptation, 156
Addiction treatment, 161, 171
ADHD (attention deficit
    hyperactivity disorder), 155–156
Adult Video News, 139
African Americans and sexually-
    oriented moral panics, 19
"Aggravated" sexting, 91
Alcohol, 136, 165
Amateur pornography, 47–48
American Ecstasy (Nitke), 45–46
America's War on Sex (Klein), 185
Anti-porn activists: communication
    with porn consumers, lack of,
    142–143; Confluence model, 136;
    experience of watching porn,
    variety of, 144–145; ideology vs.
    empirical analysis, 133–135; junk
    neuroscience, 168–169; other
    agendas, 186–187; presentations

of, 133; "rape culture," 135–136;
    on violence in pornography,
    136–140
Anti-porn industry, 31. *See also*
    Moral entrepreneurs
Anti-vaccination movement, 18
Ashley Madison hacking scandal,
    191n13
Asperger's Syndrome, 155–156
"Attachment style," 137, 154
Attention deficit hyperactivity
    disorder (ADHD), 155–156
Attwood, Feona, 141
Augustine, St., 116

Baby Doll, 11
Bachmann, Michele, 18
Backward masking scare, 18
Barry, Marion, 161
BDSM, 82
BHF (British Heart Foundation),
    163
Biblical arguments against
    pornography, 107–108

Billion Wicked Thoughts, A (Ogas and Gaddam), 38
Birth control pill, 13
Blackwell, Elizabeth, 6
"Body-punishing" sex, 138
Brain development, 28, 30, 78
Brash Films, 43–46
Braun-Harvey, Doug, 153
Breasts, 48
Bridges, Ana, 139
British Heart Foundation (BHF), 163
Broadband Internet. *See* Internet
Brownmiller, Susan, 134
Bundy, Ted, 26
Bush, George H. W., 14
Bush, George W., 12–13, 21

Cañon City, Colorado, 93
Carnes, Patrick, 30, 161
Carpenter, Bruce, 167
Cashmere, Damian, 45
Catholic Church: child sex abuse, 190n4; contraception, 14; HIV/AIDS epidemic, 13; public health critique of pornography, 26
Causation, 169–170
CCA (Comics Code Authority), 18
Celebrities: comparing ourselves to, 53, 54, 67, 80, 111; "sex addiction," 161
Centre for Addiction and Mental Health, 136
Child abduction, 18
Child pornography: adult porn not a gateway to, 181; Deep Web, 23; discussion of, 1–2; misinformation and myths, 29; progression to, 194n3; sexting and, 89, 93–94
Child sexual exploitation, decreasing rates of, 33
Children, and pornography. *See also* Sexting: brain training, 78; communication and, 76; confusion, potential areas of, 81–82; early sexualization, 79;

feelings of guilt or shame, 82–83; future sexual relationships, 78; inaccurate ideas about sex, 80; masturbation, 83–84; misinformation and myths, 77–80; molestation, 78–79; opinions of women, 78; "porn addiction," 79; porn literacy checklist, 85–86; secrecy and, 75–76; sex information websites for kids, 181–182; sexual problems, 80
China, technological change in, 20
Citizens for Community Values, 21
Cleopatra, 40
Clergy. *See* Counselors
Clinton, Bill, 14–15
Coercion, depictions of, 139–140, 144–145
Collecting pornography, 127–131
Comic books, 18, 19
Comics Code Authority (CCA), 18
Communication: about sex, 105–106, 183, 187; through pornography, 123–126
Communications Decency Act, 45
Concerned Women for America, 25
Concussions, 187
Condoms, 6, 13
Confluence model, 136
Consent: ethics of, 96; sexting and, 90–92, 95–96
Contraception, 14, 19
Contrasting labels of issues, 26–27
Counselors: avoid references to what's normal, 178–179; clients' porn literacy, increasing, 180; counseling vs. politics, 180; dealing with addiction issues, 179; differential diagnosis, 178; encourage couples to talk about sex more than pornography, 183; guidance for talking about pornography, 177–178; healthy porn use, definition of, 182;

increasing porn literacy and sexual intelligence, 175–183; meaning of pornography, 179; other issues involved, 182–183; PornPanic and, 181; sexual information and kids, 181–182; taking sides, 178; use of porn vs. desire for partner sex, 180–181; values around masturbation, infidelity, and lust, 178

Couples' conflicts about pornography: biblical arguments, 107–108; collecting pornography, 127–131; communication through pornography, 123–126; competing with women in pornography, 111–112; curiosity and empathy, need for, 57–59; demands vs. collaboration, 102–105; example of, 115–121, 123–126, 127–131; innovative approaches to, 99–113; other issues involved, 143–144; pornography use as infidelity, 106–107, 115–121; power struggles, 108–110; therapists' approaches to, 100–101; therapists taking sides, 112–113; understanding the problem before problem solving, 102–106; unspoken grievances, 102–103

Couple's contract, 100–101, 106–107

Couples therapy, 99–113. See also Couples' conflicts about pornography

Curiosity, in relationships, 57–59

Current Sexual Health Reports, 162

Deep Web, 23

Defense of Marriage Act, 14, 18

Delegitimization, 143

Desire, vs. fantasy, 38–39

The Devil in Miss Jones, 45

Diamond, Mickey, 52

Differential diagnosis, 178

Digital natives, 89

Dines, Gail, 135, 136, 138, 142, 144, 192n6

Disruptive technologies, 13–16

Divorce, decreasing rates of, 28, 33

Dobson, James, 26

Dopamine, 168

Douglas, Michael, 14, 161

DSM-5, 162, 179

Dungeons & Dragons scare, 18

Dworkin, Andrea, 21, 134

Edwards, Jonathan, 191n11

Elders, Joycelyn, 18

Emotional pain, 3

Emotions, regulation of, 152

Empathy, in relationships, 57–59

Erectile dysfunction, 163–166, 168, 198n17

Erection problems, 29, 80

Erotic power play, 65–66

"Experimental" sexting, 91

External pressure, 150

Extramarital affairs, 169

Family Research Council, 25

Fantasy. See Sexual fantasy

Fear of judgment, 153–154

Female sexual passion, 28–30, 66–68, 144

Feminism, 2, 26, 66, 144–145

Fetish, 48

Fifty Shades of Grey, 29, 38, 101

Filtering software, 21, 191n15

Finkelhor, David, 87–88, 94

First Amendment, 12

Fisher, William, 137

Focus on the Family, 26, 33

Funk, R.E., 140

Gay pornography, 61–62

Girls & Sex: Navigating the Complicated New Landscape (Orenstein), 92

GoAskAlice.columbia.edu, 85
Goodyear, Charles, 6
Government studies, 134
Graham, Sylvester, 83
Green, Laci, 182
Greer, Germaine, 17
Guilt, feelings of, 82–83
Gutenberg type, 189n1

Hartley, Nina, 45–46
Hasinoff, Amy Adele, 90
Herdt, Gil, 17
HIV/AIDS epidemic, 13, 18
Homosexual obsessive compulsive
    disorder (HOCD), 169
Homosexuality, fear of, 14, 18
Hostile masculinity, 136
Hughes, Donna Rice, 134
"Hypo-reactivity," 169

ICD-10, 179
Immorality campaign, 11–12
Immorality critique of pornography,
    19, 25–26
Impeachment, 15
Impersonal orientation to sexuality,
    136
Infidelity, 14; masturbation as
    a form of, 107; pornography
    use as, 27, 106–107, 115–121,
    141
Internal pressure, 150
Internet: attempts to censor, 14;
    changes in viewing pornography,
    7; as a disruptive technology,
    13–16; introduction of, 12–13;
    mental stimulation from, 165;
    overuse of vs. overuse of porn,
    181; results of pornography
    being available via, 15–16;
    role of, 189n3; use, growth of,
    19–20
"Internet addiction," 150–151
"Internet Gaming Disorder," 150
Internet predators, 21

Intimacy, 29
Intimate relationships, curiosity and
    empathy in, 57–59

Jensen, Robert, 134, 135, 140,
    192n6
Jeremy, Ron, 46
Johnson, Eithne, 133
Johnson, Lyndon, 134
Journal of Sex Research, 135
Judgment, fear of, 153–154
Juvenile Law Center, 94

Kazan, Elia, 11
Kellogg, John Harvey, 83
Kennedy, Anthony, 190n6
Kerner, Ian, 164
Kinsey, Alfred, 19, 62
Kinsey Scale of sexual orientation,
    62
Knapton, Mike, 163
Komisaruk, Barry, 167
Kramer, Andrew, 164

Lady Chatterley's Lover, 189n2
Law, sexting and, 92–97
Lawrence v. Texas, 12, 190n6
Legion of Decency, 11
Lesbians, and sexual fantasy, 40
Levick, Marsha, 94
Low-brow novels, 6
Lowe, Rob, 161

MacKinnon, Catharine, 66, 134
Malamuth, Neil, 136, 137
Malden, Karl, 11
Manson, Charles, 18
Marie Antoinette, 40
Marijuana, 165, 193–194n18
Marijuana scare, 18
Masturbation, 18; advantages of, 84;
    as an emotionally safe alternative
    to partner sex, 154; erectile
    dysfunction, 165–166; feelings
    of guilt or shame, 83–84; as a

form of infidelity, 107; "porn addiction" and, 171–172; problems with, 151; uses of, 181
Masturbation panic, 19
McGraw, Phil, 109
McGuire, Rusty, 93–94
McKee, Alan, 25, 141
Media: coverage of pornography, 143; PornPanic and, 187; sexting and, 92–97
Media literacy, 69, 80–81
Meese Commission, 134
Megan's Law, 18
Men, concern over personal involvement with pornography: definition of a porn problem, 156–157; emotions, regulation of, 152; erotic conflicts, 153; external pressure, 150; internal pressure, 150; introduction to, 147–150; performance anxiety, 154–155; porn problem vs. Internet problem, 150–151; porn problem vs. masturbation, 151; sex-related trauma, 154–155; sexual dynamics, 151; sexual inexperience, 155–156; shame and fear of judgment, 153–154; using porn to mediate other problems, 151–156
Mental health professionals, 22. See also Counselors
Misinformation and myths, children and pornography, 77–80
Mitchell, Sharon, 46
Mixed-gender fantasy, 62
Molestation, 78–79
Monogamy, 106–107, 116
Moore's Law, 87, 193n2
Moral entrepreneurs, 17–18, 25. See also Anti-porn activists
Moral panics. See also PornPanic: about pornography, 20–21; effect of on couples' assumptions about pornography, 101–102;

examples of, 18–19; introduction to, 17–18
Morality in Media, 21, 25, 135–136
Morals, changing roles of, 11–12
Morgan, Robin, 134
Morin, Jack, 153

Narrative, controlling, 26–28
National Center on Sexual Exploitation, 136
Neuroscience, 27, 30, 166–170
Nicotine, 163
Nitke, Barbara, 45–46
Nitke, Herb, 45
Nixon, Richard, 134
No-Fap, 168, 172
Northwestern University Law School, 135
Nylon, 189n1

Objectification, 67
Older people in pornography, 40–41, 48
Oppression Paradigm, 133, 142
Orenstein, Peggy, 92
Orgasm: in *American Ecstasy*, 46; collecting pornography and, 156; communication about, 183; during film shoot, 45; as the goal of sex, 64; masturbation and, 54, 120, 151; neuroscience, 167; in partner sex, 81; in pornography, 29, 86, 180; and pornography, myths about, 169; pressure to produce, 156; women and, 70
Oz, Mehmet, 164

Pachard, Henri, 45
Pacific Center for Sex and Society, 135
Parental relationships, 155
Parents Television Council, 25
Partner sex, 63–64, 153–154, 197n2
Paul, Pamela, 134
Penthouse, 12

Perfect bodies, myth of, 47–49

Performance anxiety, 154–155

Performances, consumption of, 67, 111–112

Pfaus, James, 165, 167

PIED (Porn Induced Erectile Dysfunction), 27, 163–164

Planned Parenthood, 17–18

Playboy, v, 5, 12

Polysemicity, 144

Popular culture, ideas of what is normal and, 109–110

"Porn addiction": in counseling, 103–104, 148–149; counselors, advice for, 179; definition of addiction, 159–160, 162–163; diagnostic criteria, lack of, 197n1; DSM-5, 162; erectile dysfunction, 163–166; evidence against, 170; fallacy of, 159–173; invention of, 27, 30; masturbation and, 171–172; myth of, 79; neuroscience, 166–170; as part of PornPanic, 170–172; partner sex and, 197n2; popular culture and, 109; symptoms vs. non-addiction explanations, 172

Porn Induced Erectile Dysfunction (PIED), 27, 163–164

Porn literacy, 69, 85–86, 175–183

Pornhub, 40

Pornography: concern over personal involvement with, 147–157; cultural ambivalence, 177; decreasing rates of certain social problems, 28, 33; definition of, 2; as demeaning to women, 27, 65–68, 138–139; effect of on consumers, 133–145; empirical evidence concerning, 133–135; as a form of infidelity, 106–107, 141; gender differences in using, 29–30; going to a porn shoot, 43–46; history of, 11–16; as a job, 44–45; lessons from, 69–71; as a

means to learn about sex, 15; mechanics of vs. meaning brought by consumer, 43–44; misinformation and myths, 28–30; misuses of, 22–23; narrative of as a dangerous product, 26–28; vs. partner sex, 80–81; religious groups on, 191–192n1; secrecy and, 29; as a threat to marriage, 27; typical content of, 28; variety of bodies in, 47–49; violence vs. nonviolent content, 28–29; watching vs. partner sex, 63–64

Pornography consumers: anti-porn activists, 133–140; caricatures of, 143; Confluence model, 136; difficulties that aren't about porn, 143–145; men's satisfaction with partners' bodies, 141–142; violent content, effects of, 136–140; voices of, 141–143

Pornography industry, and the Internet, 7

PornPanic: concern over personal involvement with, 150; counseling professions and, 181; definition of, 19; definition of a porn problem, 156–157; effect of on couples' assumptions about pornography, 101–102; effects of, 185–186; examples of moral panic, 18–19; exploitation of, 21; features of American society and, 21–23; introduction to, 16, 17–18; media and, 187; misinformation and myths, 28–30; "porn addiction" as part of, 170–172

Pottery, 189n1

Power dynamics, 65–66

Power struggles, 108–110

Presley, Elvis, 19

Privacy, changing nature of, 90

Private vs. public behavior, 26

Production Code, 6
Professional football, 187
Public health critique of
    pornography: anti-porn activists,
    135–136; controlling the
    narrative, 26–28; effect of on
    couples' assumptions about
    pornography, 101–102; effects of,
    185–186; vs. immortality critique,
    19, 25–26; introduction of,
    25–26; misinformation and
    myths, 28–31; Utah legislation,
    31–32

"Rape culture," 135
Rape jokes, 195n12
Rape/rapists, 2, 135–136, 140,
    195n14
Reagan, Ronald, 134
RebootNation, 168
"Reduced sensitivity," 169
Registered sex offenders, 191n8
Reid, Rory C., 167
Reisman, Judith, 191n10
Robinson, Marnia, 168
Rock 'n' roll music, 19
Rough sex games, 82
Royalle, Candida, 46
Rubber, 189n1
Rule 34, 51–52

Same-gender fantasy, 61–62
Satanic ritual abuse, 18
Savage, Dan, 17, 154
Scalia, Antonin, 190n6
Scarleteen.com, 85, 182
Scientific studies: erectile
    dysfunction, 165; lack of, 186;
    lack of impact on debate, 143–
    145; neuroscience, 166–170; on
    pornography consumers, 141–143;
    sexual violence, 135–137,
    139–140
Seduction of the Innocent (Wertham),
    18

Self-esteem, 32, 55, 142, 177, 178,
    183
Sex, etc., 182
"Sex addiction," 14, 30, 161, 169,
    197n4
Sex education, 13, 14, 15, 18, 187
Sex games, 139–140
Sex Plus, 182
Sex toys, 7, 82, 126
Sex trafficking, 21, 23, 28, 171,
    198n30
Sex-related trauma, 154–155
Sexting: activists on, 88–89; adult
    feelings about, 88; "aggravated"
    sexting, 91; as child pornography,
    93–94; consent, 90–92;
    introduction to, 87–88; media
    and legal responses, 92–97,
    194n20; parental advice, 95–97;
    potential criminal charges, 89–90;
    potential problems, 89–90;
    sexual double standard, 92;
    social disapproval, 89–90;
    typologies of, 91
Sexual dissatisfaction, 14, 28, 29
Sexual double standard, 92
Sexual fantasy: vs. desire, 38–39;
    feelings of guilt or shame, 82–83;
    gay pornography, 61–62; lesbians,
    40; limitless of, 51–52; meaning
    of, 38–39; nature of, 37–41; older
    women, 40–41; as a predictor of
    behavior, 179, 194n3; preferences,
    39–40; teens and, 40; variety of,
    40–41
Sexual inexperience, 155–156
Sexual intelligence, 175–183
Sexual orientation, 61–62, 169
Sexual self-esteem, 55
Sexual violence, 21; decreasing rates
    of, 28, 33, 135–136, 140;
    misinformation and myths, 30;
    scientific studies, 135–137,
    139–140
Sexualization of children, 79

Sexually-oriented moral panics, 18–19
Shame, feelings of, 82–83, 153–154
SIECUS, 182
Silvera, Joey, 46
Smartphones, misuses of
    pornography and, 22–23
Snuff films, 18
Social change, 20
Social problems, decreasing rates of,
    28, 33
Spellman, Francis Cardinal, 11
Starr, Kenneth, 15
Starr Report, 15
Stoltenberg, John, 66, 134
Stripping/strippers, 144
Suicide, decreasing rates of, 33
Sullivan, Ed, 19

Taboo eroticism, 153
Tattoos, 89
Tavris, Carol, 166
Technological change, 20, 189n1
Teen pregnancy, decreasing rates of,
    28
Teen sexting. See Sexting
Teens, 40
Therapists. See Counselors
Thought vs. behavior, 194n1
Training, lack of for clinicians, 22
Trueman, Patrick, 21
Tyler, Meagan, 139–140
Tyson, Mike, 161

Unintended pregnancy, 14
University of Arkansas, 14
University of Hawaii, 135
Unspoken grievances, 102–103
U.S. Department of Justice, 12, 21,
    135
Utah legislation, 31–32

Viagra, 154, 165
Violence. See Sexual violence
Violent content, 137–140

Weitzer, Ronald, 133
Wertham, Fredric, 18
Westboro Baptist Church, 18
Whisnant, Rebecca, 66, 138, 144
Williams, Tennessee, 11
Wilson, Gary, 168
Winfrey, Oprah, 109, 134, 161, 178
Withdrawal symptoms, 160
Women. See also Feminism:
    competing/comparing with
    women in pornography, 53–55,
    111–112; demeaning, 27, 65–68,
    138–139; opinions of and porn,
    78; self-esteem, 142
World Health Organization, 179

XXXChurch, 168

Young adult fiction, 193n11
YourBrainOnPorn, 168

About the Author

DR. MARTY KLEIN has been a Licensed Marriage & Family Therapist and Certified Sex Therapist for 35 years—that's 35,000 sessions with men, women, and couples, working on various relationship, intimacy, and sexual issues.

Klein is the award-winning author of seven books, published in 15 languages. He appears frequently in the national media, including *The New Yorker*, *The New York Times*, *20/20*, *The Daily Show*, and National Public Radio. He is outspoken about many popular and clinical ideas about sexuality; for example, he is recognized by Wikipedia as one of the most important voices in America's controversy about "sex addiction."

An internationally respected expert in the use and impact of pornography, Klein serves on the founding editorial board of the *Journal of Porn Studies*, is a contributor to the Pornography section of *The International Encyclopedia of Human Sexuality*, and has testified in court cases on the subject across the United States and internationally. A sought-after lecturer, he also recently gave two Congressional briefings on evidence-based sex education.

His monthly electronic newsletter, *Sexual Intelligence*, goes to 7,000 subscribers; his *Psychology Today* blog has an even larger following. His popular blog and website (www.SexEd.org) are frequently cited as sources of innovative thinking about sexuality, culture, politics, and the media.

CPSIA information can be obtained
at www.ICGtesting.com
Printed in the USA
BVHW040308220119
538320BV00001B/1/P

9 781440 852213